FOULKEWAYS

The Treasure and The Dream

A Message From
Gwynedd Monthly Meeting of Friends
To Residents at Foulkeways
January 1967

Foulkeways at Gwynedd carries out a dream of Gwynedd Friends Meeting which began when a neighbor (not a Friend) left a beautiful farm to the Meeting for use as a memorial to his wife May Foulke Beaumont. After much consideration the Meeting concluded that such a memorial could be created best if the farm were used to accomodate a community planned for older citizens where every feature of the architecture and the services could be designed especially for their needs; where facilities could be provided to meet every health hazard without disrupting family and friendly ties, where activities could be made available with their special interests in mind, but most of all where people could find persons of common interest and comparable age with whom to share the mature friendship and mutual support that only the rich experiences of a lifetime make possible.

To the future residents of Foulkeways
Gwynedd Meeting gives with love
its treasure and its dream

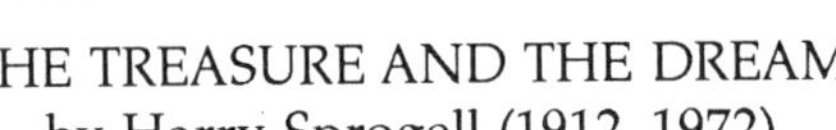

THE TREASURE AND THE DREAM
by Harry Sprogell (1912–1972)

FOULKEWAYS:

THE TREASURE AND THE DREAM

by

Blanche Perkins Zimmerman

Photographs by

Donald Birtley Brant

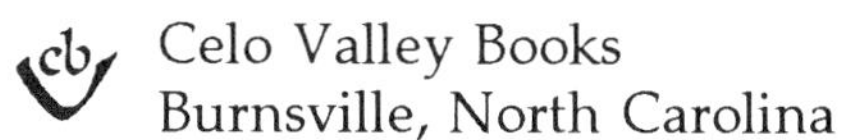

Celo Valley Books
Burnsville, North Carolina

This book can be ordered by contacting:
Foulkeways at Gwynedd
1120 Meetinghouse Road
Gwynedd PA 19436
Telephone: 215/643-2200

Line drawing of Japanese bridge by Douglas A. Tweddale.

Library of Congress Catalog Card Number 92-71095
ISBN 0-923687-17-3.

To all those whose hard work helped to bring the dream to reality, but especially to

Helen G. Stees

for her constant efforts with the Beaumont property from the day it came to Gwynedd Meeting to the present day, and to

C. Edward Zimmerman

for his suggestion that the ground be used for a place where aging, retired people could live productive lives in comfort and security in the midst of beauty and peace, and for his continual support throughout the writing of this history.

CONTENTS

(continued)

LIST OF PHOTOGRAPHS

In addition, there are four full-color insert sections.

PREFACE

"Something good must come out of Gwynedd Meeting," Eliza Foulke once said at a Meeting for Worship. "Gwynedd Meeting is so richly blest, something good must come out of it."

And so it has. It is almost certain that neither the committee which began the process which resulted in Foulkeways, nor the hard-working individuals who ushered in the final phases of its creation ever suspected that they were fulfilling a prophecy. But they were since, sometime later, Foulkeways came out of Gwynedd Meeting.

What follows is the story of life as it is lived and managed at Foulkeways at Gwynedd, the first Continuing Care Retirement Community (CCRC) in Pennsylvania. Members of the Religious Society of Friends (Quakers) administer this eminently successful and financially secure endeavor.

Foulkeways is located in the township of Lower Gwynedd, Pennsylvania, just twenty miles north of Philadelphia and one mile from the commuter rail line to the city. It is a place where the physical, intellectual, psychological, and spiritual needs of the aging are met in creative and productive ways. This is reflected in the atmosphere of well-being and happiness which is evident at Foulkeways.

This history is based on the records of Gwynedd Meeting, of the Board of Directors, of the Foulkeways Residents' Association, and on conversations and observations of those who live in the Continuing Care Retirement Community called Foulkeways.

— *Blanche P. Zimmerman*
Foulkeways, January, 1992

ACKNOWLEDGMENTS

I am indebted and exceedingly grateful to:

Donald Brant, for his excellent photography and his enthusiasm. He has taken pictures all over the world and shares them in travelogues. He took all of the pictures in this book with the exception of the two portraits, the aerial view, and a few in part one which were taken by early residents. His enthusiastic support has been invaluable.

Gwynedd Mercy College, where my whole life was expanded, and to my wonderful friends there, especially one of my professors:

Anne Kaler, who always pushed me beyond myself, for her criticism and encouragement;

Sydney Hunt, who encouraged me to reach beyond Foulkeways and who helped me to do so;

Margaret Jacques, for just everything;

Lelage Kanes and Donald Schwartz, who advised and corrected me on commas, composition, and consistency;

Richard Willis, who lived through the creation of Foulkeways, and who corrected the accuracy of my reporting;

Bertram Zumeta, for his specific recommendations.

I also owe a debt of thanks to:

The Board of Directors of Foulkeways, the Foulkeways Residents' Association, and to Marion Price, for their generous financial help;

The Friends Historical Library at Swarthmore College, for making the records and minutes of Gwynedd Friends Meeting available to me;

The Administration of Foulkeways, for allowing me access to their records, and especially to Brenda Ware and Dorothy Frank for their help and unfailing patience.

Special thanks go to Diana Donovan of Celo Valley Books, for her sensitive copyediting and expert guidance.

I have no advice for thee. All that I can say is if thee is on the right track, the way will open.

— James B. Walker

PART ONE

The Treasure and the Dream

THE TREASURE

Eliza Foulke was not very happy when her lawyer husband, Thomas A. Foulke, was called out on the stormy night of October 16, 1945 to go to the home of Charles O. Beaumont to prepare a will. Although the Beaumonts lived just across DeKalb Pike from Gwynedd Meeting, the two men had never met.

Thomas, never one to shirk an appeal, collected his materials and went out into the storm. He was astonished, as he laid out his papers, to hear Charles Beaumont say that he was going to leave his property in Lower Gwynedd Township to Gwynedd Meeting to honor the wishes of his late wife, May Foulke Beaumont. Thomas's surprise was sharpened by the fact that the Beaumonts were members of the Episcopal Church of the Messiah, a stone's throw down DeKalb Pike from Gwynedd Meeting. They had never been inside Gwynedd Meeting and, as far as anyone knew, they had no interest in the Society of Friends. When informed of the will, the members of the Church of the Messiah must have been surprised also, as were some cousins who, no doubt, had expected to inherit something from the Beaumonts.

Mr. Beaumont was familiar with death. His wife, May, and their two children, Mason and Gwen, all had died within the previous six years, leaving him with no heirs. He may have had a premonition of his own impending death, for he died on November 25, only forty days after he had signed his will. Had he died within one month, the will would have been invalid.

May Foulke Beaumont was from the same rootstock as Thomas Foulke. Their common ancestor was Edward Foulke who, with his wife and nine children, arrived in Philadelphia back in July 1698. They were members of the Welsh Company which had sent William John and Thomas Evans ahead to the New World to select and purchase a site for a settlement in William Penn's new grant from King Charles II of England.

There had been four Evans brothers among the original Welsh purchasers. And the Beaumont property was part of the Evans' grant signed by William Penn's deputies. (The sheepskin on which that grant was written has been framed and now hangs in the Beaumont parlor at Foulkeways — a gift from the Horace G. Evans family.)

A pamphlet, *Gwynedd Monthly Meeting of the Religious Society of Friends, 1699 - 1949*, relates:

> The advance agents had chosen well — a fertile, wooded land of peaceful valleys and gentle hills, high in elevation and watered by the Wissahickon and Treweryn Creeks. It is not known who named the tract, but the word "Gwynedd" [pronounced Gwyneth in Welsh] means the "white land" and symbolizes the pure and beautiful, the untaken virgin country. (p. 5)

In the historical chronology of the property (see Appendix C) "Gwynedd" is defined as meaning "high ground." Both high ground and white land were applicable.

According to the pamphlet, May Foulke's grandfather, Dr. Antrim Foulke, a member of Gwynedd Meeting and a great-great grandson of Edward Foulke, purchased the property from its original builder in 1823. As was the custom then, May Foulke may have been "read out of Meeting" when she married Charles Beaumont, because he was not a Friend. We know that she was not, herself, a member of the Society of Friends when she died. But she had a strong affection for her grandfather, and she wanted Gwynedd Meeting to have his cherished homestead because she knew of his love for the Meeting.

Thomas Foulke electrified Gwynedd Meeting when he announced at the December 1945 monthly meeting that just before Charles Beaumont died he had willed the nearby property to the Meeting with no restrictions for its use, other than that it serve as a memorial to his wife, May Foulke Beaumont. The property consisted of a large and imposing house which was furnished with antiques, a doctor's office, another smaller house with some furniture in it, a small barn, and sixty-four acres of farmland with a larger barn on it across Meetinghouse Road. Although the property would not legally be turned over to the Meeting until the will was settled, there were some things, such as taking care of the furniture in the two houses, which needed to be done immediately. The executors of the will graciously permitted the Meeting to proceed as though it were the deeded owner from the time of the announcement of the death of Charles Beaumont.

At the January 1946 monthly meeting, a Beaumont committee was appointed to begin to evaluate the situation and set some priorities for action. Those on the committee were Horace G. Evans, chairman, Helen G. Stees, secretary, Thomas A. Foulke, Eliza A. Foulke, Russell E. Paton, Helen M. Price, Harry E. Sprogell, John A. Stees and Marguerite I. Wolf as members.

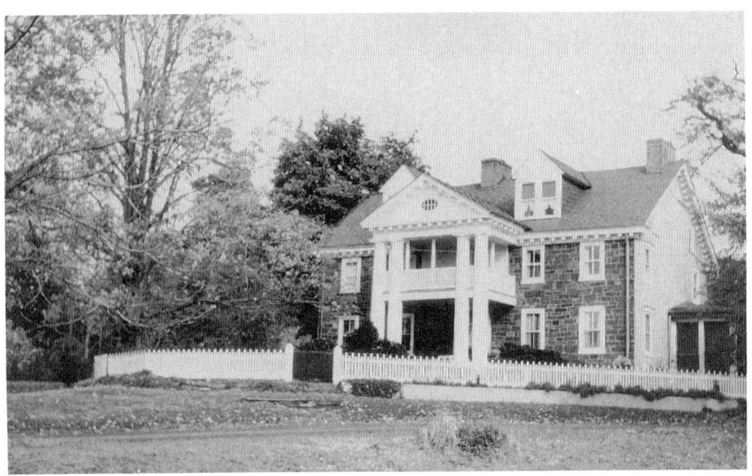

Beaumont House

When the Meeting received the news of Mr. Beaumont's death, it was looking toward a building program and needed to raise $35,000 to pay for it. It was tempting to think of selling the inheritance to pay for the new addition. After sober reflection, however, the Meeting staunchly determined that it would not be appropriate to use the proceeds from the sale, or make any use of the property, to meet Gwynedd Meeting's needs. On the other hand, the Meeting would not use funds contributed by its members to pay taxes or upkeep of the newly-acquired property. The two entities would remain separate. Ways must be found to get funds needed for the Beaumont property until some definite use of the new real estate could be agreed upon.

The antiques in the big house at the junction of DeKalb Pike and Meetinghouse Road were the first concern of the committee. As many of them as could be used were saved to furnish a room at the Meetinghouse, which was then called the Beaumont Room. (These things were eventually put into the Beaumont parlor at Foulkeways as a focus of the memorial to May Foulke Beaumont.) A fine old grandfather's clock was repaired, restored and placed in the East Room of Gwynedd Meeting. A good piano from the smaller house was repaired, tuned, and put into service at the Meetinghouse.

It took the Meeting more than a year to make and implement the decisions about the contents of the two houses. Those things not suitable for a sale were disposed of in various ways. Finally, in February 1947, a public sale was held. Proceeds from the sale — amounting to $3,867 — plus several contributions, brought the May Foulke Beaumont Memorial Fund (which had been established to receive contributions) to $4,591.

This concern for the furniture was accompanied by a desire to have the houses occupied. The rent would provide the committee with needed money, and tenants would help keep the buildings from deteriorating in the way empty houses do. Notices asking for suggestions for use of the houses for the summer of 1946 were put in the *Gwynedd Newsletter* and also in the *Friends Intelligencer*, a Quaker weekly in Philadelphia.

As a result of the notice in the *Intelligencer*, a request came from the Bedford Center in Philadelphia for a place in the country where it could bring inner-city children for the summer. The Bedford Center was a Philadelphia Neighborhood Center on Kater Street in South Philadelphia which worked to improve the lot of the area's residents. After consulting the executor of the Beaumont estate, the zoning board, the road commissioners of Lower Gwynedd Township, and a sampling of the neighbors, the monthly meeting in May 1946 authorized the Beaumont committee to proceed with plans for the Bedford Center to use the smaller house (called the Lowry house).

Some repairs had to be made before the group, which hoped to occupy the house from May 15 to September 30, could be accommodated. The roof needed repairs; water, electricity, and plumbing had to be installed. Money from the May Foulke Beaumont Fund was used for these improvements. The rental for the summer was one dollar.

The Bedford Center had a very successful summer. The Lowry house was a good place for the children. It was away from DeKalb Pike traffic and there was the barn for rainy weather play. There was also ample space for gardening which was a major activity of the children. In a report to the monthly meeting in August, the Beaumont committee reported that the Bedford Center occupants had cleaned up and put the Lowry house in much better condition than they had found it. Indeed, they may actually have saved the Meeting some costly repairs. The boys slept in the attic and the girls and the two counselors occupied the second floor. One night the boys, terrified, woke up the counselors screaming, "The ghosties be clickin' they teeth." The counselors comforted and reassured the boys, then went up to the attic with them to sleep. Sure enough, as soon as they were settled, they heard what sounded exactly like teeth clicking. This was reported to Helen Stees, the liaison person from the Beaumont committee. She immediately called an exterminator who discovered that the clicking noises were caused by powder post beetles. They had already done considerable damage and could have ruined the whole structure had they not been discovered.

There was still the problem of getting the Lowry house in better condition and finding tenants for the winter. Heat had to be provided before the cold weather set in. The committee agreed to put in the heater, and then try to find a young couple in need of housing who could live there, rent-free, from October 1, 1946 until June 1, 1947. The tenants would be responsible for any improvements they wanted to make.

The committee was happy to report to the Meeting in November that Stephen and Mildred Thiermann would be

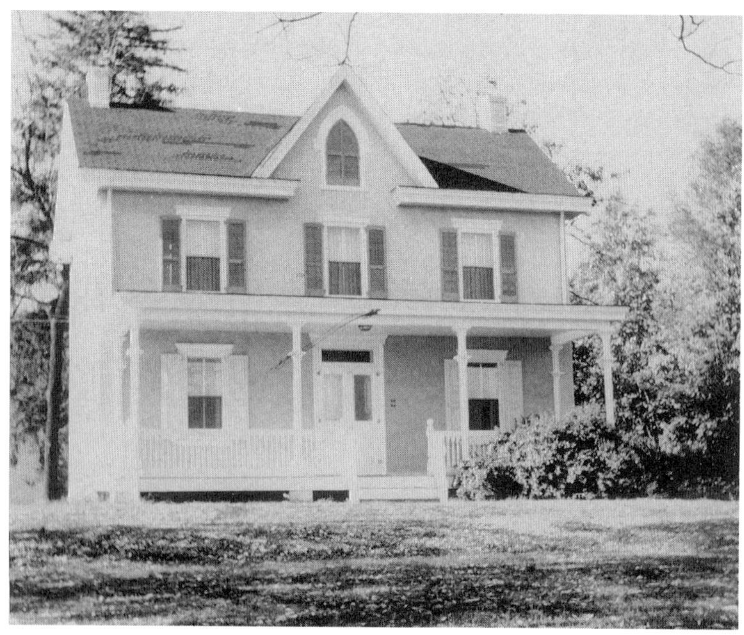

Lowry House

living in the Lowry house for the winter. Stephen, a conscientious objector during World War II, had just finished working in the Philadelphia State Hospital and was now with the American Friends Service Committee.

The monthly meeting in February 1947 was a busy one. Thomas Foulke reported that the Beaumont estate had been settled and Gwynedd Meeting was now the deeded owner of the Beaumont property. With characteristic understatement, the clerk of the Meeting recorded that "the Meeting approved the acceptance of the bequest of Charles O. Beaumont." The minutes went on to record that "Friends heartily approved the donation to Thomas Foulke of letters patent from the Commissioners of William Penn to Edward Foulke, found among the family papers of the late Charles O. Beaumont."

The Beaumont committee announced that the Beaumont house was being leased to two young couples, the Bartons and the Sandersons. These conscientious objectors would share the whole house, and would pay the Meeting $100 per month. The rent was less than might otherwise be obtained, but the Meeting was sure it would be more than compensated for any monetary difference by the contributions these tenants would make to the life of the Meeting.

Also at the February meeting the Beaumont committee was thanked for its assiduous work in handling all the details pertaining to the Beaumont property. Both houses had been emptied of their contents and the Thiermanns were settled in the Lowry house. The committee was released from service and the trustees of the Meeting assumed the responsibility of the property from then on. One of the first things the trustees did was make plans to convert the Beaumont house into two apartments as soon as it was feasible. The house was large enough to make two nice-sized apartments, which would be easier to rent than one large house.

The Thiermanns were the first of a parade of fine young couples to occupy one or the other of the two houses from the time they moved in during the fall of 1946 until after Foulkeways was built. Some of the others who lived there were the Baers, Byrds, Hartsoughs, Hoskins, Osterkamps, Reads, and Martin Truebloods, all of them with young children. In 1951 Doris B. and Edwin S. Jones, older, very active members of the Meeting, moved into the Lowry house. They lived there until Edwin died in 1969 and Doris continued to stay until she moved into Foulkeways in 1972. Harry Sprogell reported to the monthly meeting for the trustees at one time, "the greatest value of the property to date has been the great strength that those who have lived [in the two houses] have brought to the Meeting."

The farm acreage was another matter. It had not been farmed for some time and the soil was as poor as could be found anywhere in the county. When it was wet the clay soil was impossible to get through with a plow, and when it was dry it was as hard as a rock. The top soil was very thin and what there was had been washed down to the several hedgerows which crossed the land. In fact, the top soil was so thin that the early residents of Foulkeways thought that it had been skimmed off and sold.

It was desirable to have the land under cultivation, since untended land rapidly grows up in weeds, brambles, and saplings. The last effort to farm it, sometime in the 1950s, had resulted in complete failure. Edward Zimmerman, a farmer and member of the Meeting, looked at it with an eye to cleaning up the ground but soon found it to be too big an undertaking. So the ground was left to lie open and unused during those years when the Meeting was trying to decide what to do with it.

At some time during all the considerations about the Beaumont property, Thomas Foulke became aware of a piece of ground which bordered the farmland and fronted on Sumneytown Pike. He suggested to Gus Martin, then President of the Trustees of Gwynedd Meeting, that the Meeting should buy this piece of property so as to provide an outlet onto Sumneytown Pike. It took two or three monthly meetings of earnest discussion before there was unity in the Meeting and the ground could be bought. This was accomplished in March 1951, and was a boon for the future of Foulkeways.

From 1946 to June 1953, many suggestions for a proper use of their inheritance were discussed among Gwynedd Meeting members. Some of these suggestions were: a retreat center, a community library, a conference center similar to Pendle Hill, a Friends school, a summer camp for the needy, housing for conscientious objectors, and low cost housing for others, especially the elderly. Some wanted to sell the property and use the proceeds for education scholarships for the young people of the Meeting. Although all of these suggestions were duly considered by the Meeting, most of them never reached the committee stage and those which did were short-lived. One by one, they were rejected for one reason or another. The one constant in all the explorations was that there must be a fitting memorial to May Foulke Beaumont.

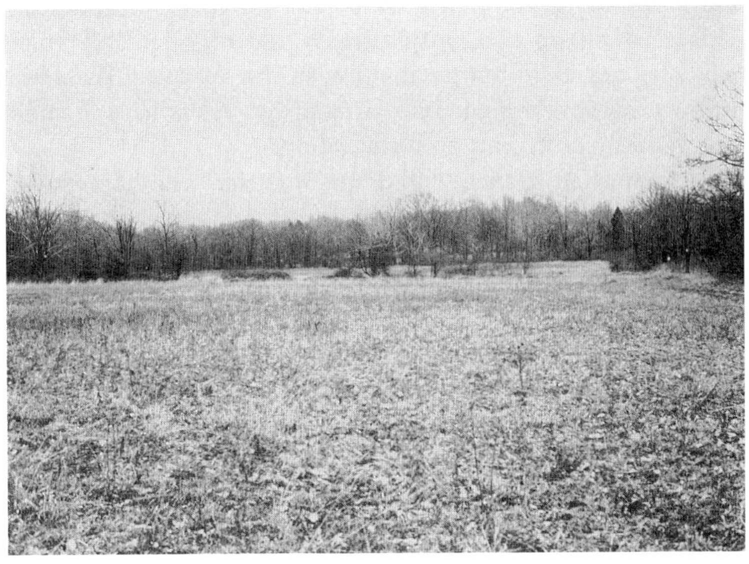

Beaumont Farm before Foulkeways (looking south)

The suggestion which made the greatest impact on the Meeting was the one which culminated in the formation of the homesteads committee. This group's activities began in the fall of 1946, even before the property was officially turned over to the Meeting, and continued until the committee was dissolved in 1953.

Mark T. Deibler was the first chairman of the twenty-seven member committee. The committee reported to the monthly meeting from time to time over a period of six or seven years, and it seemed, finally, that this was something the Meeting could unite on. To make a fitting memorial for May Beaumont and a significant contribution to Gwynedd Meeting, as well as be a credit to the community of Lower Gwynedd Township, their hope was to establish an integrated community for socially concerned families.

When Edward B. Peacock, chairman of the homesteads committee, reported to the Meeting in April 1953 that the committee was ready to go and, if the Meeting approved, would begin to sell lots to prospective builders, the committee received a shattering blow. A "weighty" (influential) Friend stood up and, with sorrow and regret in his voice, said that he could not go along with the proposal. As is well known in Quakerism, one dissenting voice in a Quaker business meeting can stop an action.

A shocked silence wilted the Meeting. The homesteads committee was summarily laid down. A member was heard to say that it looked as though, by default, *nothing* was ever going to be done with the Beaumont property. Another wondered whether Charles Beaumont had had his tongue in cheek when he directed the writing of his will. Had he said to himself, "Let's just see how these good Quakers with all their patience and good works will handle this?"

With the homesteads committee now discontinued, the initial enthusiasm of Gwynedd Meeting members for their inheritance was deflated. In its last gasp the homesteads committee reminded the Meeting that it had a moral responsibility to do something, "at least in a small way to meet our obligation" to make a proper memorial according to the will. The committee suggested that a project to plant small evergreens might be undertaken, stating that a donation of a few thousand such trees had been offered.

Nothing came of the tree-planting idea, though, and the Meeting settled down to a lethargic acceptance of the status quo of the farmland. The rents from the two houses came in regularly, which made it possible to pay the taxes and keep the houses in repair. There were times, however, when the Meeting had to help with some of the larger expenses (such as drilling a new well for each of the houses), tapping special Meeting funds to do so. Except for an occasional change of tenants all remained quiet on the Beaumont front during the next five years.

THE DREAM

As the years passed, Edward Zimmerman, a member of Gwynedd Meeting, had become more and more aware of the strain it had been on his mother when his two grandfathers lived with them for so many years. He realized it was not always the ideal arrangement for the two old men, either. He glanced around the Meeting and wondered what kind of living arrangements the older members here might be anticipating, and he looked across DeKalb Pike to the Beaumont farm.

He had an inspiration. Why not use the Meeting's inheritance to build a place where the retired and aging could live independently and happily, and where they could be taken care of when necessary?

It was more than five years after the homesteads committee had been discontinued when, in October of 1958, Edward Zimmerman suggested to the monthly meeting that the Beaumont property be used for a "cottage type" retirement community for the aging. In typical Quaker fashion, a committee was appointed to explore the possibilities of such a community. Those appointed to serve on this new Beaumont committee were: Wilbert L. and Nina P. Braxton, Paul W. and Esther S. Goulding, Harry E. and Barbara S. Sprogell, Arnold E. and Caroline F. Trueblood and C. Edward and Blanche P. Zimmerman.

Edward Zimmerman was asked to be chairman of the committee and Blanche Zimmerman agreed to serve as secretary. The committee was asked at this time to consider also whether a portion of the land might be used for a school. There is nothing further about a school in the monthly meeting minutes. If it was ever considered, it was not recorded.

The original minutes covering the five years of activity of this new committee were later condensed into less than two pages of recorded notes. These two pages were bound in the minute books of Foulkeways and the originals were discarded. As a consequence, this section of *Foulkeways: The Treasure and the Dream* is based on the monthly meeting minutes of Gwynedd Meeting and the personal recollections of those involved.

The newly-formed committee began its responsibility with an open field before it — both literally and figuratively. There was no other retirement community in the area to serve as a guide; new ground would be broken. What was visualized was a completely new concept of a way of living for the retired and aging. The committee members had never heard the phrase "continuing care" but that was what they were after. They never deviated from the idea that there should be complete care, covering every aspect of daily life from the day of entry until death.

The dream from the very beginning was that there should be three stages of living offered in the new community: independent apartment living, an intermediate stage of living under supervision, and skilled nursing care in a separate facility. Three meals a day were to be served in a central dining room and there would be as many amenities as possible for the physical, intellectual, emotional, and spiritual well-being of the residents.

Those on the Committee talked of their dream at every opportunity: at Quarterly Meetings and Yearly Meetings, with weighty Friends, with residents and management of existing Friends' Homes, with township officials and, indeed, with anyone who would listen. The first detailed report to the monthly meeting in March 1959 shows the great enthusiasm of the committee, as recorded in the monthly meeting minutes:

> Everywhere we have found encouragement and enthusiasm — from those for whom such a possibility has come too late, to those who would welcome such

> an opportunity now, and those who are looking ahead. We are convinced that this is a great and growing need, becoming more urgent as the life span increases.
>
> The Meeting was satisfied with the report of the Committee and gave approval for further exploring and planning. It was willing to have the matter discussed with Abington Friends Home in Norristown, since it was aware that some changes appeared to be in the offing for that Home and there might be an area for cooperation there.

The committee very quickly became aware of the need to hire an architect to give direction to its nebulous thinking and talking. Arnold Trueblood suggested that Robert Venturi, a gifted young architect with the firm of Venturi, Cope & Lippincott, be asked to work with it. Robert Venturi agreed to develop a plot plan and floor plans for a fee of $2000. There was no budget in the monthly meeting for this committee, but the Meeting agreed to underwrite the expenses until money could be found.

At the monthly meeting in May 1959 the addition of John A. and Helen G. Stees to the committee was approved. The committee warmly welcomed John and Helen. In one way or another they had been involved with the Beaumont property from the time the Meeting inherited it.

There is nothing from the Beaumont committee in the monthly meeting minutes from May 1959 until March 1960. The committee members had not been idle, however. They had hired Robert Venturi and he had made plot plan drawings and designed and built a model of an apartment building containing four apartments. Neither the plot plan nor the model building bore much resemblance to what was eventually built. Nevertheless, as a tangible and graphic start, the plan gave the committee members something to show, talk about and hang onto as their thinking evolved toward the actual development of their dream. The model was shown at Gwynedd Meeting, at Quarterly Meeting in Norristown and it was on display in the East Room of the Arch Street Meetinghouse all during Yearly Meeting. A

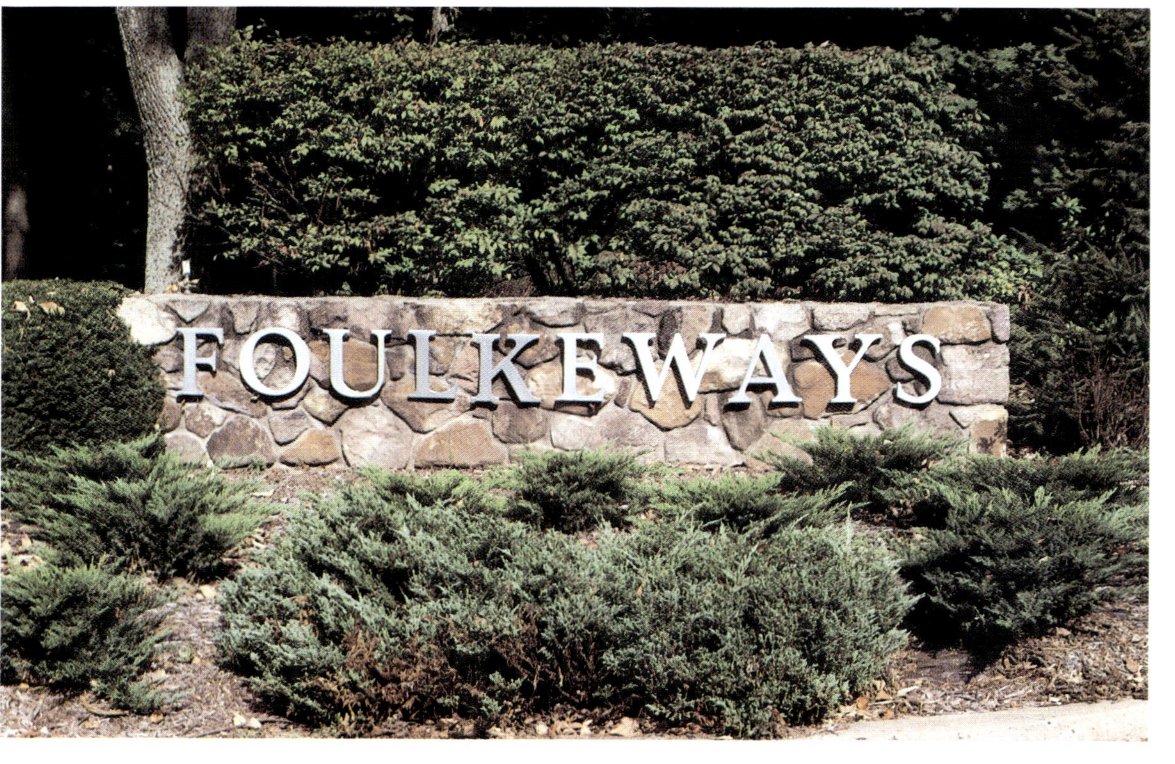

Entrance to Foulkeways off Sumneytown Pike

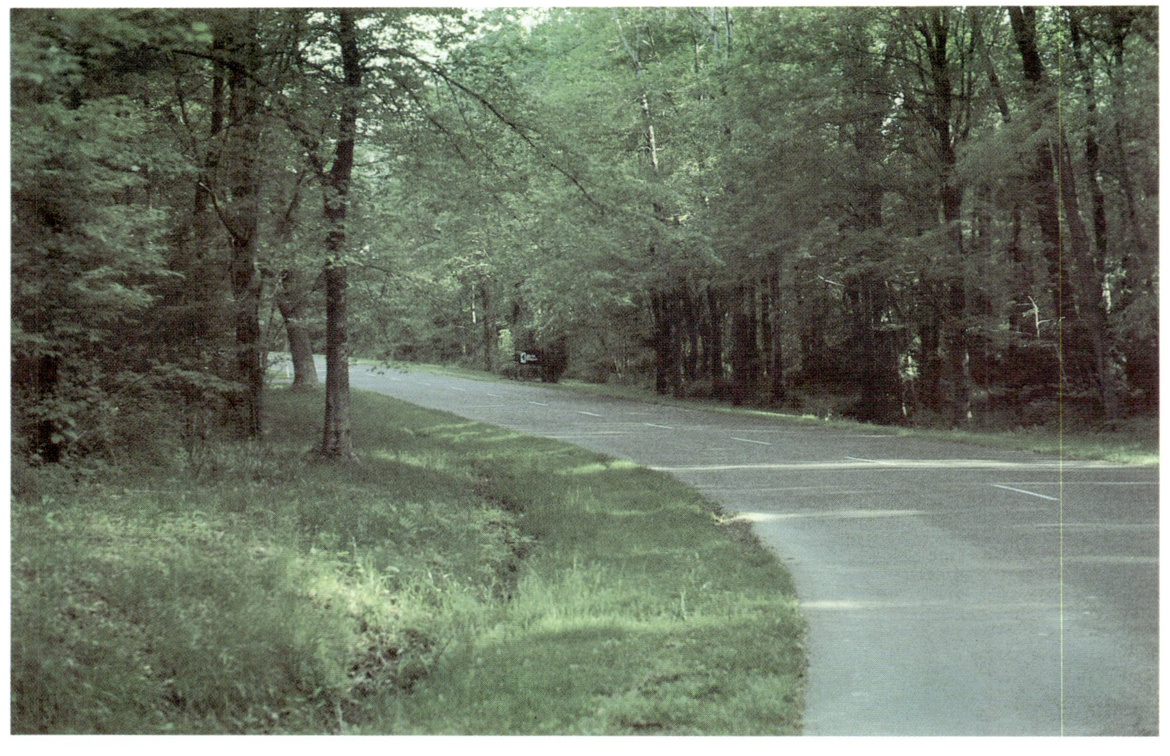

Perimeter Road

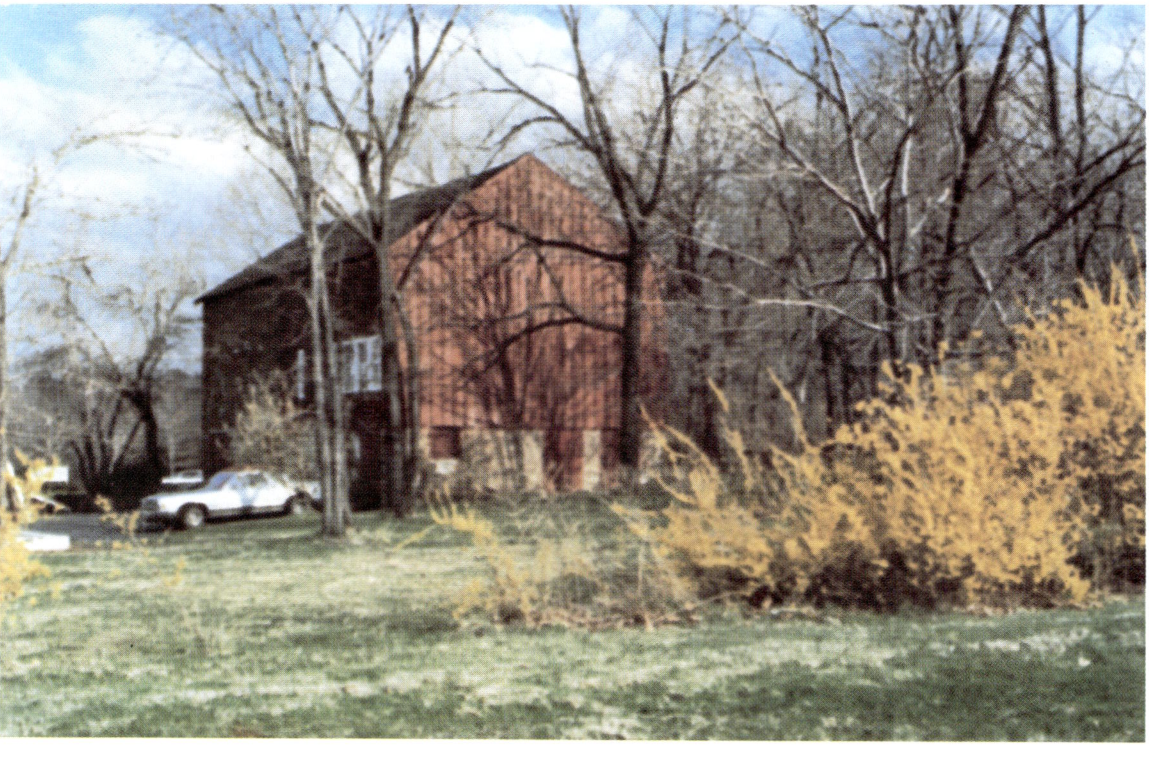

Pennsylvania Bank Barn

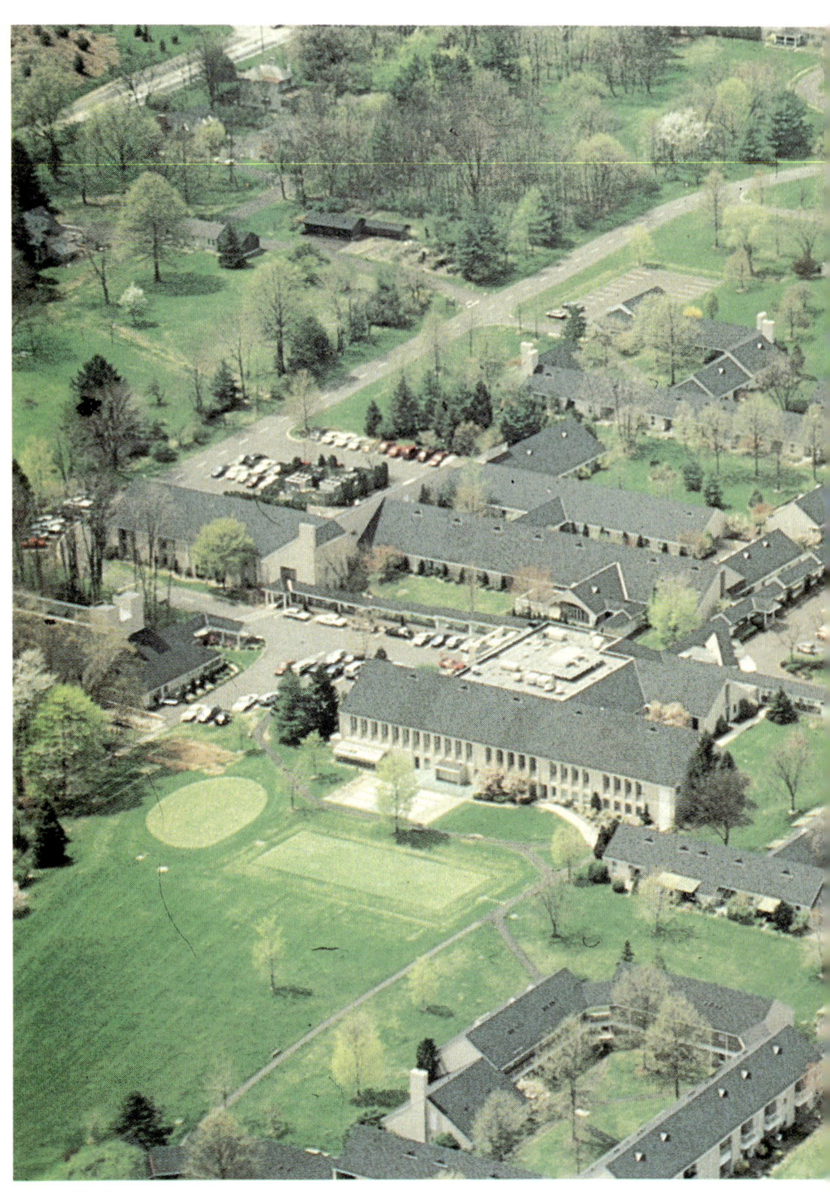

Foulkeways at Gwynedd, Meetinghouse Road, Gwynedd PA 19436.

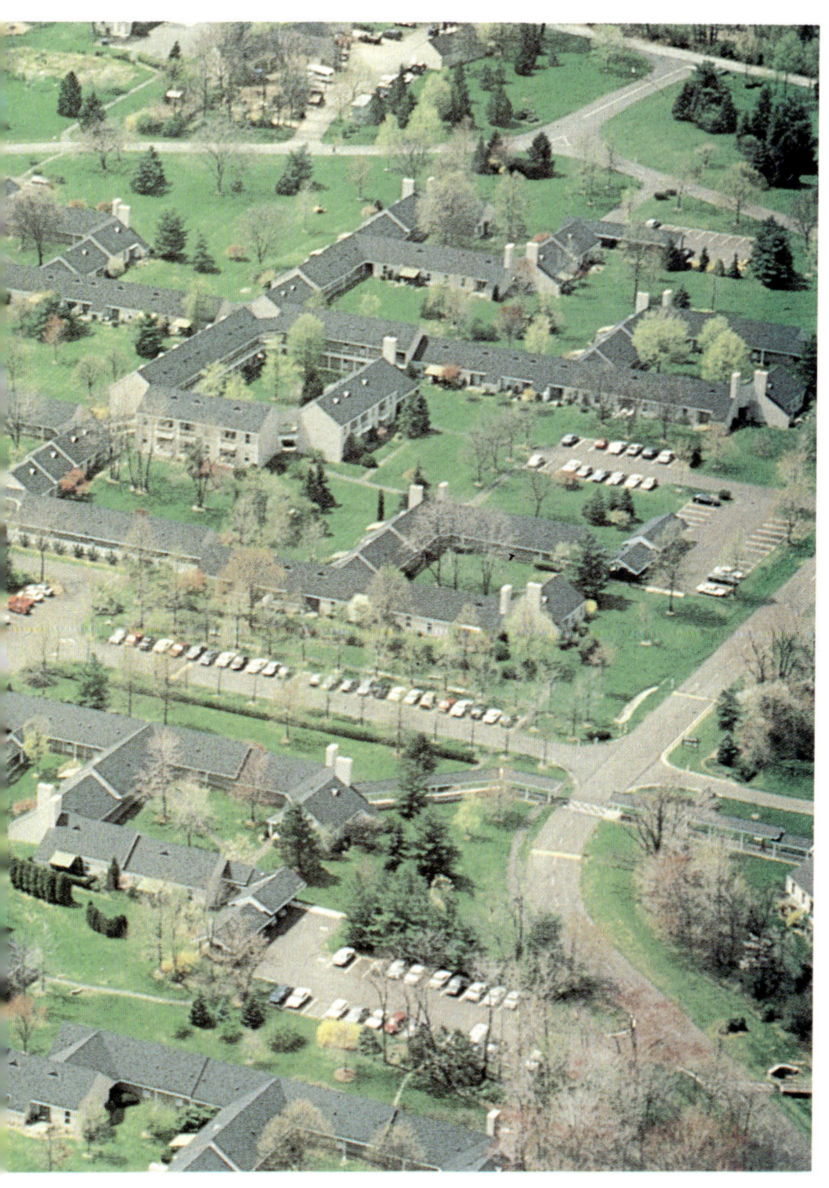

Aerial view of the campus of Foulkeways, looking north.

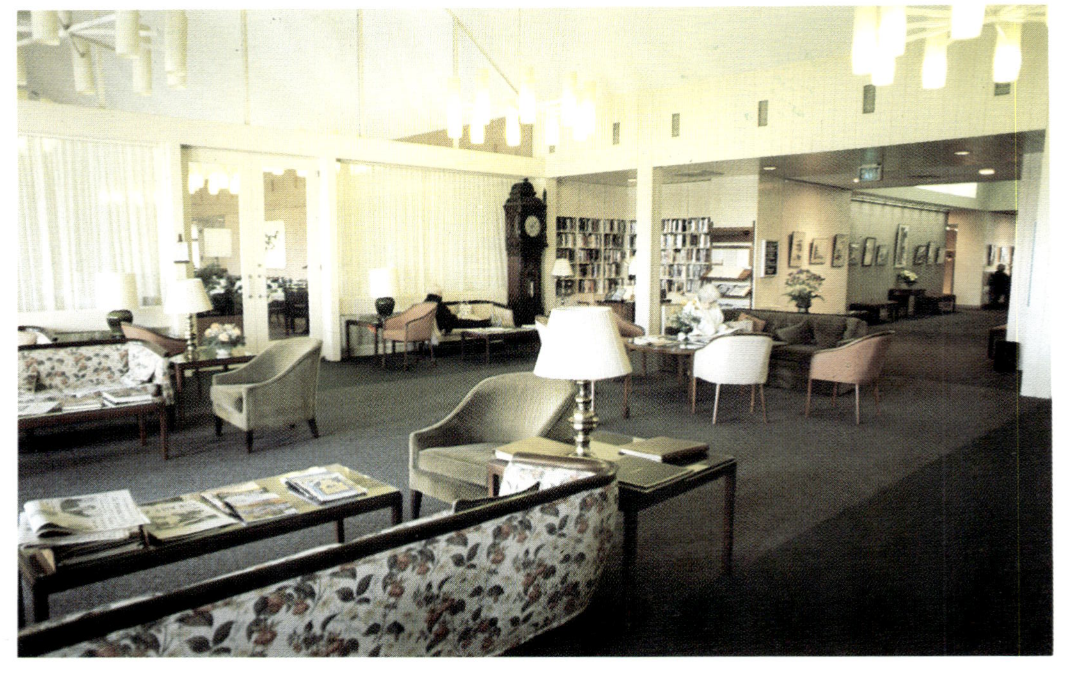

Lobby in Central

Main dining room to left; auditorium to right.
Pictures by local artists changed monthly.

Main Dining Room

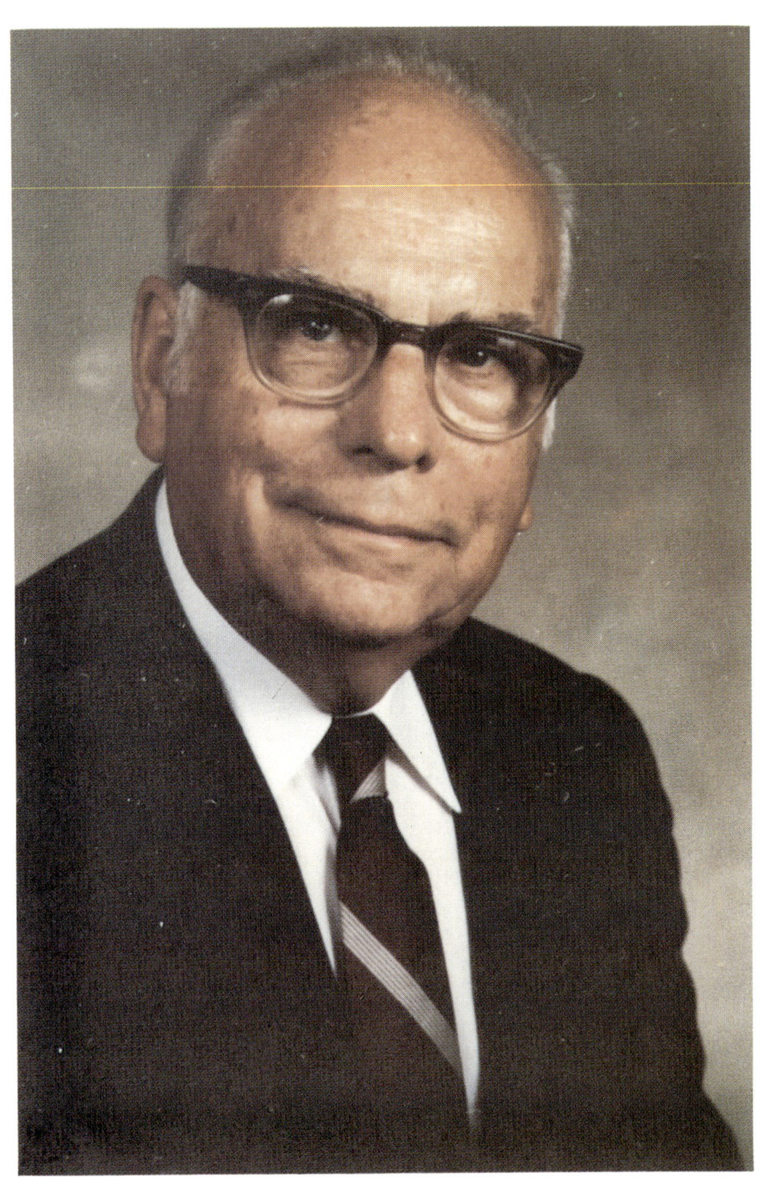

Allen J. White
1911–1989
First Executive Director, Foulkeways

member of the committee was always on hand to explain the plans and answer questions.

The Shoemaker Fund was asked for a grant of $1,000 which was approved. This, along with contributions of $200 each from Paul Goulding and Edward Zimmerman (this is mentioned here only to correct the erroneous report in the condensed minutes that these two men had each contributed $1,000), was applied to the architect's bill leaving a balance of $600. There is no further mention of funds for the Beaumont committee in the monthly meeting minutes, but the bills got paid by contributions from persons interested in the idea.

The committee reported to the March 1960 monthly meeting that the name of Foulkeways, suggested by Paul Goulding, had been chosen for the future community. The Meeting was pleased with this choice because it left no doubt about the projected retirement center's being a memorial to May Foulke Beaumont.

In October 1960, a meeting was held at the Meetinghouse to which all the neighbors, as well as some other interested persons, were invited. There was a gratifying amount of interest shown. Even though many questions were asked, no objections to such a community in the area were heard.

Nothing seemed to be standing in the way of moving ahead, yet nothing was really happening. There was no progress. There was a sudden recognition by the committee members that the exciting plans were becoming stalled on dead center.

Excerpts from a lengthy report which John Stees made to monthly meeting in February 1961 are interesting, for they outline almost exactly what was eventually done. They are the result of a meeting which John Stees had with the chairman of the Lower Gwynedd Planning Commission. Included were the following statements:

> Although the Lower Gwynedd Supervisors and Planning Commission are favorably inclined to the Foulkeways concept, no permit for construction will

> be approved until local, county and state requirements for sewage disposal are included in the plans. Just what these will entail will require definition by the County Planning Commission and the State Board of Health.
>
> The next obvious step is to continue working with the Lower Gwynedd Planning Commission to develop a satisfactory sewage disposal plant. ... Assuming that plans for sewage disposal are acceptably developed the next series of steps is:
>
> a. Gwynedd Meeting should dissolve the present committee and establish a non-profit corporation which should have full power and discretion to finance, build and operate the Foulkeways project. The corporation man-power should not be limited to Gwynedd members, but should enlist from Yearly Meeting dedicated Friends with special talent and experience in organization, finance, construction and multiple-housing management who can and will devote the time needed for such a project.
>
> b. After the formation of the corporation, Gwynedd monthly meeting should cede and transfer all right, title and interest in the Beaumont land to the corporation.
>
> c. Further development of financing, construction and operation should be the full responsibility of the corporation, free and clear of Gwynedd Meeting.

What held up progress at this point? Who knows? The report of the Beaumont committee to monthly meeting in May 1961 reflects to a great extent the contents of the Stees report, and also the lack of movement within the committee. That report begins: "For over two years the Beaumont committee has met, dreamed, planned, hoped — and muddled." The committee asked for and received permission to appeal to Representative Meeting for advice and support. Representative Meeting referred the matter to Friends Hall, a facility in Philadelphia for caring for "confused, elderly Friends." Nothing was heard from either group. Also at that May monthly meeting, the committee lost as members,

Paul and Esther Goulding. Paul had made arrangements to attend the Earlham College School of Religion in Indiana, so they were released.

More than two years had now elapsed since the idea of a retirement community was first proposed to Gwynedd Meeting. A stultifying feeling of discouragement had seeped into the minds of the committee members, yet no one was able to analyze the problem. In retrospect, it is easy to see where the trouble lay. No one on the committee had any notion of whether or not a project such as it was proposing would work. No one had seen or heard of such a retirement community. The committee was facing a daunting proposition with unknown consequences, and there did not seem to be any driving imperative to convince any of the group to assume such a risk. Another angle which is obvious in hindsight is the fact that the committee seemed to be waiting for someone to come forward, pick up the idea and run with it. As an exasperated Friend said when he was approached the second time for advice, "If you people out there at Gwynedd want to do something, *you'll* have to do it. There is nothing I can do for you."

From time to time during those months of frustration a prominent Friend would be invited to come to the Meeting for Worship on First-Day, then to dinner at the home of one of the committee members. James B. Walker, a longtime Headmaster of Westtown School, along with his wife, Alice B. Walker, was one of these. When the plans were laid before him and his advice asked, his reply was, "I haven't any advice for thee. All I can say is that if thee is on the right track, the way will open."

The way did not seem to be opening. Perhaps the committee was on the wrong track.

Frank A. Libbon was welcomed to the committee in the spring of 1961. He was a bit older than the other members and was eager to see Foulkeways become more than mere words and fruitless meetings. He went to Washington, D.C. to the office of the Federal Housing Authority to see about getting a low-interest loan. A person from the FHA came to

Gwynedd, walked over the ground, surveyed the surrounding area and decided that this was no place to put a retirement facility. It was too far out in the country, too far from shopping, too far from transportation, too far from cultural activities, too far, just too, too far. "What do you think you have to offer people?" he asked before refusing help.

The committee accepted this refusal stoically. No one agreed with all of his objections and moreover, the FHA would have imposed more restrictions than the committee cared to contend with, had it borrowed money from them. Yet it did dampen the already low spirits of everyone.

At one of the meetings it was decided to put a notice in the *Friends Journal*, the successor to the *Friends Intelligencer*, briefly outlining the plans and inviting anyone who might be interested to join the group. Harry Sprogell had been absent when that decision was made, and when he heard that it had been carried out he was not very happy.

"No, no, no," said Harry. "You can't tell who might answer and we'd have to take them whether we wanted them or not." But the committee was fortunate. The only response that came was from Norman and Gertrude Winde, the same Norman Winde who was later president of the Foulkeways board of directors from February 1965 until May 1975.

There is nothing about the Beaumont committee in the monthly meeting minutes from June 1961 all through 1962 and up to January 1963. A general apathy had settled over the members of the committee. No meetings were being held, no leadings were appearing, no encouragement or stimulation came from any quarter. It looked as though this idea for the use of the Beaumont property was going the way of all the others — simply fading into oblivion as just one more notion which fell through for the use of Gwynedd's treasure. All of the showings of the model, all of the talking, planning and hoping — everything had come to nought.

The dreams had been enchanting, but it had finally become apparent that the dreamers were not able to bring them into existence. In the group were a successful lawyer, an award-winning builder, two leading educators, an experienced engineer, a successful businessman and a master farmer — all experts in their respective fields, plus their accomplished wives. Yet they either did not know what steps to take to set the plans in motion, or they did not have the time or energy for such a huge undertaking. What was sorely lacking was a forceful imperative, an igniting spark to set the thing off. The secretary decided to call a meeting of the lifeless committee to recommend that it be discontinued at the January 1963 monthly meeting.

However, early in January 1963, not long before monthly meeting, Dorothy N. Cooper, a consultant for an ad hoc committee of Philadelphia Yearly Meeting on the Care of the Aging, called Blanche Zimmerman, the secretary of the Beaumont committee. Dorothy had seen the model and the plot plans created by Robert Venturi which had been on exhibit at Yearly Meeting, and she had heard a little about the dreams of the Beaumont committee. Dorothy Cooper was working on her annual report to the Yearly Meeting on the care of the aging and wanted to include in her report whatever it was that Gwynedd Meeting was doing, or was planning to do, about Foulkeways. Could she meet with someone to talk about it?

She was told that the beautiful dreams were just that — beautiful dreams and nothing more and it would be a waste of her time to come. She insisted that she wanted to hear about it anyhow, so she drove out from Philadelphia to meet with Barbara Sprogell and Blanche Zimmerman. As she listened to what was being told to her, Dorothy Cooper grew more and more excited. "You have *got* to find a way to do this," she exclaimed. "There is such a great need for exactly what you have outlined here. You *must* do it." Was this the missing imperative?

Instead of calling a meeting to consider having the

committee dissolved, the secretary, after consulting with the other members of the Beaumont committee, spent the time writing out a detailed report of the meeting with Dorothy Cooper for the January monthly meeting. In it she told of Dorothy Cooper's great enthusiasm for the idea of a retirement community and of her insistence that it be done. The Meeting was asked to name new members to the Beaumont committee and to give permission for the Beaumont committee to recruit members from the Yearly Meeting membership.

There had been some vague rumors that someone was interested in buying the property. In view of all of the above, the Meeting was asked to refrain from selling the Beaumont house and triangle, including the Lowry house, for a period of six months, and to give the committee permission to become incorporated. The Meeting gave its approval to all these requests.

Those persons from Gwynedd Meeting who were added to the Beaumont committee at this time were: Lorraine W. Deibler, Joseph S. Evans II, Martha P. Hankin, Warren N. Helman, August L. Martin, Marion W. Martin, Ann L. Osterkamp, W. Russell Stott, Richard B. Willis, and Lowell E. Wright.

As a result of the meeting with Dorothy Cooper and the subsequent monthly meeting decisions, Barbara Sprogell and Blanche Zimmerman went to the Yearly Meeting office in Philadelphia where Francis G. Brown, General Secretary of the Philadelphia Yearly Meeting, allowed them to go through the membership files in their effort to enlist Friends for an enlarged Beaumont committee. From the Yearly Meeting files they compiled a list of names of about one hundred persons, which they divided among the members of the Beaumont committee.

All those on the list were called and asked if they would be willing to work on the project. Eleanor Stabler Clarke's name was on the list. When she was called her reply was, "You don't want me. You want my husband, Bill. He's the one in our family who knows about these things."

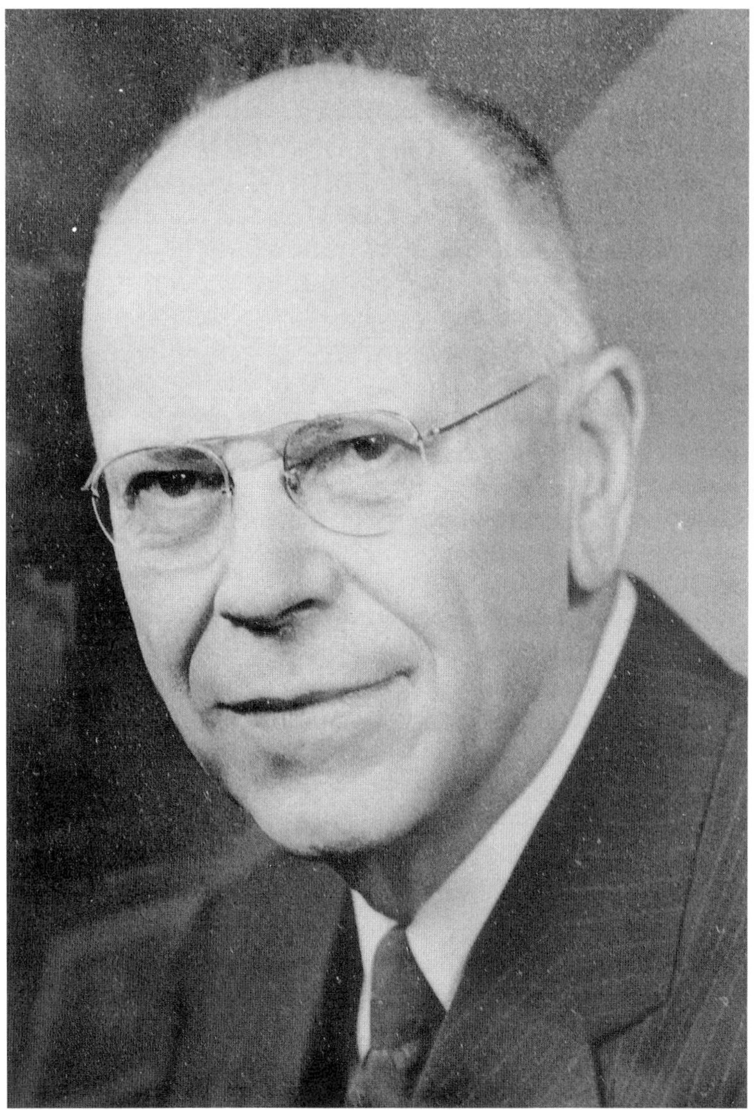

William A. Clarke
First President of Foulkeways
January 31, 1896–February 8, 1965

William A. Clarke agreed to work with the committee on the project, as did Allen J. White and some fifty other persons. They were all invited to come to a Meeting for Worship at Gwynedd on April 28, 1963, after which there was a luncheon prepared by members of the Gwynedd group, followed by a meeting of the Beaumont committee.

Harry Sprogell, the lawyer on the committee, was asked to chair the meeting. He described the projected retirement community which had been in gestation for five years and opened the meeting for discussion. After a few questions and answers about the possibility and feasibility of building such a community, William Clarke stood up and said, "Of course it can be done, and we will do it." Wonderful, wonderful words.

William Clarke had recently returned from a visit with a cousin who was living in a life-care retirement community in Palo Alto, California. He had seen firsthand the many advantages of such a place and was delighted to discover that plans for building one in the Philadelphia area were struggling to come into being.

The "imperative" had come from Dorothy Cooper's urgency, and now William Clarke struck the "igniting spark" which was needed to start the action: "Of course it can be done, and we will do it."

For the rest of 1963 there are only minor references in the monthly meeting minutes regarding the project. In January 1964 a report of the Beaumont committee was made. It included the following:

> After many meetings and much searching by the enlarged committee some conclusions have been reached and the next steps anticipated. ... The conclusions are that there is a real need for the kind of living facilities for older people which are being planned and that it is possible and feasible to meet these needs. ... It is estimated that it will take from two to three years to reach the point of ground breaking.

Except for a brief report to the monthly meeting in June 1964, that was the end of the Beaumont committee although it was never laid down. It finally evolved into Foulkeways at Gwynedd, Incorporated.

Beginning with the momentous meeting of the enlarged group on April 28, 1963 at Gwynedd Meeting, the Foulkeways project began to develop a life of its own apart from the Meeting. An organization committee, consisting of Frederic E. Benton, William A. Clarke, Thomas W. Elkinton, Harry E. Sprogell, John A. Stees, Allen J. White and Richard B. Willis, met early in May in Harry Sprogell's office which was in the law firm of Saul, Ewing, Remick & Saul in Philadelphia. William Clarke acted as clerk of this loosely organized group, and Harry Sprogell was the secretary.

The immediate activities of this body had to be centered on getting the necessary zoning variance from Lower Gwynedd Township. This meant getting an architect's preliminary plot and building plans, guaranteeing water and sewer access, and finding the money to pay for it all. The committee was loath to spend a large amount of money for an architect if there was any danger of not getting the zoning variance, yet plot plans were a prerequisite in the application for zoning.

Robert Venturi was asked to put together a tentative plot plan to present to the Lower Gwynedd Zoning Commission for its reaction. Gus Martin, John Stees and Ed Zimmerman studied the water and sewer possibilities and met formally and informally with the Lower Gwynedd officials. The township did not express approval, but this sub-committee reported that it felt the authorities were receptive to the idea of a retirement community on the Beaumont property and would respond favorably at the proper time.

With this encouragement, the organization committee

began to feel more comfortable about going ahead, although it remained aware of the tension involved in bringing everything together in the proper sequence. This committee reported to the overall membership of the Beaumont committee on June 26, 1963 that "future steps in prosecuting the Beaumont project would involve a very delicate balance of breadth of progress, cost of operation and other factors."

Plans were made to capitalize on the talents of the large group which made up the Beaumont committee, now being called the Foulkeways Association, through the use of ad hoc committees to help with the many concerns and problems facing the organization committee. Suggestions of where an ad hoc committee might prove useful were in the fields of architecture, finance, construction, landscaping, philosophy, health, legal matters, and public relations. A special committee to build a list of prospective residents was headed by Dorothy Cooper.

Frequent meetings with the association members, held at Gwynedd Meeting after Meeting for Worship and lunch on First-Day, were attended by from thirty-five to fifty persons, plus those on the organization committee. The meetings with the larger group served both as pep rallies and as a sounding board for the hard-working organization committee, and also furnished a degree of sorely needed manpower through the ad hoc committees. Harry Sprogell reported at one meeting that "the record-keeping, transmission of information and organizational effort required in connection with the Foulkeways project demanded more man-power than is available."

While the organization committee was coming to grips with the technical problems of zoning, sewers, and loans, Dorothy Cooper was diligently tackling issues concerning future residents. During First-Day school time at Gwynedd Meeting on October 6, 1963, Dorothy reported on her activities. She told of some conclusions she had reached when she thought about the future of Foulkeways as she wrestled with problems of the aging.

Dorothy saw two imperatives needed from opening day: a nursing facility and a central building with a dining room. In the early days of exploration it was thought that the community might be built in stages, but she was emphatic in her insistence that complete care be available before anyone could move in. During all of her activities with the aging Dorothy Cooper kept a growing list of prospective residents to whom literature and progress reports were sent. Only six months after the organization committee began to function, fifty-one persons had expressed in writing their interest in a community such as Foulkeways was planning.

As a consequence of Dorothy Cooper's convincing and inspiring talk in the First-Day school, the resolution to move ahead was strengthened. At a meeting of the Foulkeways Association held in the afternoon of that same day Harry Sprogell was asked to apply to the Trustees of Gwynedd Meeting for the title clearance to the Beaumont property which would be needed when making applications for a zoning variance and building permits from Lower Gwynedd Township.

The organization committee was enlarged on October 21, 1963 by the addition of Dorothy Cooper, William Harned, Jane Potts, and Blanche Zimmerman, bringing the total to ten. It was good to have the new members as the question of which architects to use could not be delayed and the extra voices were helpful in making the decision. William Clarke felt strongly that an architect who had had experience in designing the kind of place that was wanted for Foulkeways was crucial to the success of the endeavor. The firm of Skidmore, Owings & Merrill had designed three such places in California. William Clarke had visited one of these, the Sequoias, in Palo Alto. John and Helen Stees and Gus and Marion Martin later visited another by the same firm, Carmel Valley Manor at Carmel. They had all been favorably impressed by the work of these architects.

Although he appreciated what Robert Venturi had done for Foulkeways, William Clarke, whose voice carried weight, held out for the California architects. Other members of the group expressed disappointment that Robert Venturi was not to be involved with the project, but they reached unanimity in the matter. They insisted, then, that the builder have Quaker connections. This was not hard to satisfy, for Barclay White, Jr., a Quaker and a member of the Association, accepted the job.

The matter of publicity was tackled at a meeting on December 16, 1963. To further the work of the publicity committee, William Clarke consented to work on an outline of the costs and operating procedures for such a project according to Pennsylvania requirements. This would furnish information for the committee responsible for getting the facts before the public. The basic characteristics for the desired community that the committee wanted to publicize had been honed and were now listed. One of the items read:

> Among the attractive features which the project must have are the offer of lifetime care, a program of activities and considerable stress on the attractiveness of the surroundings.

By the beginning of 1964 the plans for moving ahead began to firm up. At a meeting of the organization committee and their spouses held on January fifth at the Sprogells' home some important decisions were made. In any Quaker business meeting there is no voting. In that setting anyone may voice an opinion which will be respected, so the spouses and their suggestions were more than welcome. The realization that costs could not be cut without imperiling attractiveness, and hence salability, was accepted as a hard fact. William Clarke was authorized to discuss with the architects the arrangements which needed to be made for moving the work forward, which would include sketches and costs. Dorothy Cooper was asked to send a report of what was going on to all the members of Representative Meeting with a covering letter in which she wrote:

> The [Foulkeways] committee is willing to assume the considerable financial responsibility involved,

> since it feels there is a great unmet need for this type of independent living among older members of Philadelphia Yearly Meeting. We hope to solicit your moral support and interest in spreading information about Foulkeways throughout the Yearly Meeting.

John Woodbridge, representing Skidmore, Owings & Merrill, came on from California to meet with what was now being called the executive committee to try to work out some areas in which the local firm of Venturi, Cope & Lippincott might be engaged. This did not appear to be practical so, with regret, the local firm was retired. William Clarke, William Harned and John Stees were authorized to close arrangements with Skidmore, Owings & Merrill as architects and with Barclay White, Jr. as builder. The decision to go forward was now clinched.

A letter dated May 13, 1964 was sent to Michael Strong, Esq. directing him to begin to collect the necessary memoranda and forms in preparation for the application for a zoning variance and building permits. This entailed having available the proper services such as water, sewers, electricity and telephones. Gus Martin had accepted the assignment to secure easements for underground water, electric and gas services for the project.

Some major decisions regarding the property had to be made before a zoning variance could be applied for. Should the large Beaumont house be a part of Foulkeways or should it be sold? How about the Lowry house and the barn? After much thought it was agreed to sell the Beaumont house and retain the Lowry house and barn. Because of the size and location of the Beaumont house, the executive committee felt it could become an encumbrance rather than an asset, so it was sold. The Lowry house was kept because the ground it was on extended over to Route 202 and this might become important at some future date. The barn was on the main parcel of ground and presented many possibilities for its use.

There were a few other matters which had to be settled

before building permits would be issued. A small, frame U.S. post office sat on the north-west corner of the farmland. As the population of Lower Gwynedd Township increased it became necessary to have a somewhat larger post office. Foulkeways leased an acre of ground for $200 per year to the government for the new building, reserving the right to establish and maintain power and sewer lines which crossed the property there. Foulkeways also had to buy a small lot adjacent to the Gwynedd Meeting property for sewer lines at a cost of $1,500. This was deeded to Gwynedd Meeting. Another matter was the placing of the Sumneytown Pike entrance at the lower edge of the property. In its planning the executive committee was careful to put the entrance in the exact center of the property so as not to offend either neighbor.

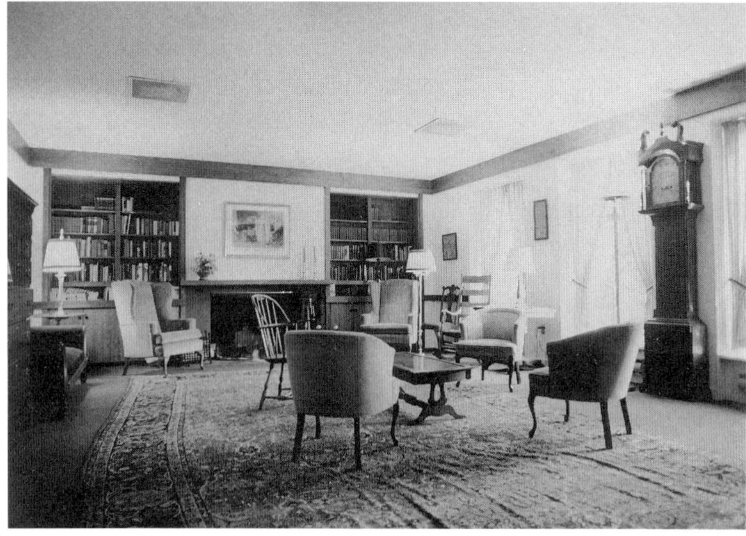

Beaumont Parlor

FOULKEWAYS AT GWYNEDD, INC.

In June 1964 a committee was appointed to bring forward an outline of a suitable corporation. Those on that committee were: Frederic Benton, William Clarke, Thomas Elkinton, John Stees, Richard Willis, and Allen White.

The certificate of incorporation was signed on August 21, 1964. The signers were William Clarke, Harry Sprogell, and John Stees. The nonprofit corporation was registered in the state of Delaware and officially named Foulkeways at Gwynedd, Incorporated. Twenty-six association members and eleven directors were elected. The corporation had the Meeting's blessing in that it had given permission to the Beaumont committee in January, 1963 to incorporate, asking only that the majority of the associates be members of Gwynedd Meeting. Twenty-two of the thirty-seven members accordingly were from Gwynedd Meeting. The following excerpt is from the minutes of the first meeting of the directors and associates of the corporation:

> The following directors were elected each to serve, (provided he continues as a member of the Religious Society of Friends) until the annual meeting of members in the year indicated or until his successor shall be named and he qualifies:
>
> 1965 — William H. Harned, Jane M. Potts, John A. Stees, Allen J. White
> 1966 — Frederic E. Benton, Thomas W. Elkinton, Harry E. Sprogell, Richard B. Willis
> 1967 — William A. Clarke, Dorothy N. Cooper, Blanche P. Zimmerman

A list of persons who were elected as additional members of the corporation is in Appendix E of this book.

The first request made to Gwynedd Meeting from Foulkeways at Gwynedd, Inc. was in September 1964. The monthly meeting minutes record:

> The Corporation requested and the Meeting approved three items:
>
> 1. The authorization to Gwynedd Trustees to join Foulkeways application for a special exemption to the zoning ordinance of Lower Gwynedd Township.
> 2. Foulkeways requested the Gwynedd Meeting Trustees to lease the Beaumont property to the Corporation for 99 years, all taxes, expenses, etc., and all liability to be assumed by Foulkeways.
> 3. Instruct the Gwynedd Meeting Trustees to execute at Foulkeways' request a mortgage on the Meeting's underlying interest in the land on the understanding that Gwynedd Meeting or its trustees will have no liability whatsoever beyond the lien on that interest.

At a meeting of the corporation members, directors, Barclay White, Jr., builder, John Woodbridge, architect, and sixteen other interested persons on Sunday, September 27, 1964, at Gwynedd Meeting the following officers of the executive committee were named: William A. Clarke, president; Harry E. Sprogell, vice-president; Thomas W. Elkinton, treasurer; Helen G. Stees, secretary; and Richard B. Willis, assistant secretary-treasurer.

Corporation members were asked to approve the action of the executive committee, to be diligent in spreading information about Foulkeways and to help locate a qualified manager. William Clarke announced that contracts had been signed with the architectural firm of Skidmore, Owings & Merrill, and he showed plot plans and room layouts which would be presented to the Board of Supervisors of Lower Gwynedd Township on the next day, Monday, September 28, 1964.

Barclay White, Jr. was introduced, and he stated that his estimate of construction time from the time of the acquisition of building permits would be from twelve to fifteen months.

At a meeting of the corporation in October 1964, Francis G. Brown, General Secretary of Philadelphia Yearly Meeting, was added to the corporation. H. Mather Lippincott, of the firm of Venturi, Cope & Lippincott, and Norman H. Winde were welcomed to the Executive Committee.

The directors were shocked and saddened in January 1965 to hear that William Clarke, prime mover and president of the board, was in the hospital, seriously ill. They also had some good news: the zoning variance had been granted by the township, almost one year after application had been made for it. The architects and builders were urged to press ahead toward securing building permits and also to work out cash flow projections and tentative costs to help in the recruitment of residents.

William Clarke died on February 8, 1965. In a minute prepared immediately following a meeting of the directors on February 15, the great loss to the board and to all those involved in the Foulkeways project was expressed:

> Through [William Clarke's] efforts the project moved from the vague to the concrete, gathering supporters as it took form. The skill of his direction will be greatly missed but the intensity of his interest will always be a standard for those who carry the project on.

Members expressed a desire that one of the buildings should bear William Clarke's name and that his widow, Eleanor S. Clarke, be invited to serve on the executive board. Norman Winde, the only person who had responded to the plea for help back in the Beaumont committee days, was unanimously elected to be the new board president.

In April 1965, exactly two years after the birth of the new life of Foulkeways, the newly-elected president announced that the operation had finally reached the point where action must begin to augment and replace talking and planning. The recently-granted zoning variance would expire in June 1966. Since construction must begin before that date, February 1966 was set as the deadline for breaking ground and starting the building.

John Fisher Smith, the project manager for Skidmore, Owings & Merrill, came to Philadelphia to review the preliminary design, budgetary estimates and arrangements for constructing the sample units. Separate zoning approval was required for the models, but this was more or less a routine matter by this time.

David H. Larson (also from Skidmore, Owings & Merrill), who had replaced John Woodbridge as the architect and whose mother, Olive Larson, later became a resident of Foulkeways, led a detailed discussion with the executive board in May 1965. The process had now come down to specifics and there were seemingly countless decisions which had to be made. It had been emphasized earlier that "the compromise between the best possible service and the lowest possible cost will be inevitable." The concern to offer a high standard of living and yet not have a "rich Quaker's establishment" which few would be able to afford, was constantly with the members of the whole group as they wrestled, planned and built. Their Quaker beliefs made it mandatory that the building be of the highest quality, built to endure. They agreed that they wanted to echo the simple architecture of the Meetinghouse for the exterior; the interior was to be designed for comfort, convenience, simplicity and beauty.

As a result of advertising, a competent manager had been found and engaged. Robert C. Trier, Jr. and his wife, Elizabeth, were introduced as a team at the board meeting in April. Before he agreed to come to Foulkeways, Robert Trier expressed his need for an assistant in the selling process. This was agreed to, as everyone was aware of the importance of the bottom line. The whole performance rested on getting fifty percent of the units sold before a mortgage could be obtained.

At a regular meeting in October 1965, Dorothy B.

Hallowell was added to the executive board. At the same meeting Thomas Elkinton resigned as treasurer, citing ill health. The board was grieved to hear at its next meeting of the death of this valued member, the second such loss within the year. Richard B. Willis, chairman of the finance committee, became the new treasurer.

The question of where and how money could be obtained arose at every meeting of the executive board. Money was needed on all sides. Preliminary architect's drawings to get proper zoning, zoning application fees, publicity costs, all these and more took money. The Shoemaker Fund gave a grant of $3,500. The Chace Fund made a loan of $10,000 to tide them over a tight spot. The Yearly Meeting later made a loan of $10,000 so the Chace Fund loan could be repaid.

As the various aspects of developing the community began to fall into place the need for "seed money" became urgent. Progress could be speeded up if enough money could be found to build the sample units which were to be used in the sales program. With the unanimous approval of the Foulkeways Corporation a letter was sent to Yearly Meeting to request a loan of $300,000 from the Eastburn Fund.

The Eastburn Fund had come to Yearly Meeting in an interesting way. Dorothy Cooper, in her capacity as a consultant for the care of the aging for Yearly Meeting, had been asked to visit Margaret Eastburn, an elderly, spinster, Quaker school teacher who was living in the Quaker boarding house at Friends Centre, Third and Arch Streets, Philadelphia.

Margaret Eastburn, in one room piled high with newspapers, magazines and other paraphernalia, was ill. She was so ill that Dorothy Cooper immediately got her into a hospital. Once settled in the hospital, Margaret expressed a desire to have a lawyer; she wanted to make her will. Dorothy Cooper smiled to herself. What did Margaret Eastburn have to will? Nevertheless, to humor the sick old lady, Alan Hunt, Esq., agreed to see her. At her request,

Alan Hunt wrote the will leaving all her worldly goods to the Philadelphia Yearly Meeting of the Religious Society of Friends, shortly after which she died. On going through her belongings, the executors of her will found securities worth around $600,000 — a fair sum in the 1950s.

One might wonder how a school teacher could amass so large a sum. She had inherited some money from a fellow school teacher, but Quaker thrift also played a part. Margaret Eastburn had lived in Atlantic City where she taught school. Every year when she went to the annual Yearly Meetings, which are held in Philadelphia, she would present a bill to the Pemberton Fund for transportation — to the exact penny. The Pemberton Fund is a fund which was set up to reimburse Friends who wanted to get to Yearly Meeting but could not afford the cost of getting there.

When Foulkeways applied to Yearly Meeting for a loan from the Eastburn Fund, it seemed entirely appropriate to lend it to a project for the aging since it had come to the Yearly Meeting through their committee on the care of the aging.

In making a financial analysis on April 25, 1965, Richard Willis explained that the board was waiting for a grant from the Chace Fund for $15,000 as well as the promised loan from the Eastburn Fund. These two items would cover certain engineering and architectural expenses and furnish funds for building the sample units. Richard Willis continued,

> We can borrow against the land, defer obligations and expect (hopefully) to receive $1,600,000 to $1,800,000 from Founder's fees on 107 units. After 107 units have been sold we can obtain a construction loan of $5,000,000. On completion, a permanent mortgage will be obtained.

This analysis was in keeping with a decision made at an earlier meeting: to ask the first generation of residents to pay half their founder's fee at the start of construction or whenever they signed up after construction had begun.

A major consideration in the planning was how to space the buildings on the sixty-four acres to the best advantage for pleasant living. Harry Sprogell reported to the corporation that:

> Rearrangement of the units has reduced the institutional aspect; using the slope of the land looking to the southeast gives a feeling of open space. There will be two units having two stories each for contrast in roof line. This will create 39–43 second-story apartments. There are persons who prefer living above ground.

With approvals for plot and floor plans out of the way and money promised, the board could begin to give much-needed attention to other matters. Stouffer's was engaged as kitchen consultants, and for food management later. Medical services were arranged with the Lansdale Medical Clinic. Resident costs had been projected and could now be verified. The founder's fees would be:

Studio unit — $9,500 - $12,000.

Living room, bedroom, bath, kitchenette — $14,000 - $18,000.

Living room, 2 bedrooms, 2 baths, kitchenette — $27,000 - 32,500.

The monthly fee was set at $225 per person.

Serious thought was given to those who might need financial assistance. There were Yearly Meeting funds which could be tapped in some cases; it was hoped that monthly meetings might be willing and able to help their own members if necessary. As a token of appreciation to Gwynedd Meeting for the gift of the ground, Foulkeways agreed to allow credit up to $28,500 for members of the Meeting. This would allow three full scholarships or various partial scholarships for an efficiency apartment.

A committee to find ways and means to help anyone

who needed assistance was set up with Allen White, Dorothy Cooper, and Eleanor Clarke as members.

A comprehensive report on "where we stand at the moment" was made to the corporation membership on November 21, 1965. There would be a total of 213 units built at a cost of $5,500,000. All of the service areas, such as the infirmary, parlors, offices, and central building facilities, were included in the time and cost estimates. Finalized plans were displayed, discussed and approved. Norman Winde, president, announced at this meeting that the project had arrived at a point where action would be required on short notice and in several areas. He appointed the following persons to serve on special committees to meet those urgent needs:

Facilities: to be responsible for contracts and definitions having to do with builders, architects, and services: Harry Sprogell, chairman, Jane Potts, John Stees, Edward Zimmerman.

Resident Recruiting: William Harned, chairman, Dorothy Cooper, Helen Stees.

Finance, Budget and Fund Raising: Richard Willis, chairman, Mather Lippincott.

Admissions and Medical Policy: Mather Lippincott, chairman, Dorothy Cooper, Eleanor Clarke.

Specific Services: To be developed.

It was necessary at this time to find a publicity agent to get out special bulletins and find creative ways to put Foulkeways before the public. Merritt Pharo, a well-qualified person, was hired for this important post. Advertisements were placed in various newspapers, especially the *New York Times* and the *Wall Street Journal*. There had been frequent items in the *Friends Journal* about Foulkeways all along and these were to be continued, as well as notices in other Quaker publications.

By January 1966 the contract for residents was shaping up. Much time, thought, and energy had gone into researching the policies of other facilities in the field, although no other project in this area offered the comprehensive program that Foulkeways was planning to have. The thought given to this contract has been made obvious by the fact that few changes have been made in it and it has served as a model for most of the continuing care communities in the Northeast.

Ground breaking occurred on April 16, 1966, some two months later than originally hoped for, and the sample units were started immediately. These model units were ready for use in early August and greatly enhanced sales as visitors began to average around twenty per day. Regina H. Peasley served as a hostess there, and Elwood P. Phillips was added to the sales force on a part-time basis. Regina's mother and future resident, Ethel K.B. Hallowell was often in the sales unit, humorously calling herself a "sample

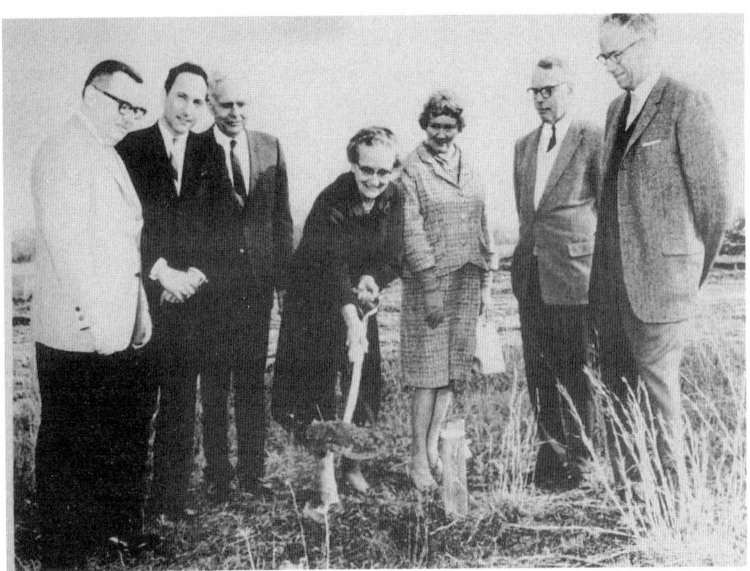

Breaking Ground

Left to right: Thomas J. Timoney, Esq., Sen. Richard S. Schweiker, Norman H. Winde, Eliza A. Foulke, Helen G. Stees, Richard B. Willis, Harry E. Sprogell.

resident." It was a great comfort to the board at this time that Robert Trier could report that the sales situation was well in hand.

The board rejoiced in June when Richard Willis announced that the First Pennsylvania Banking & Trust Company had agreed to a twenty-five-year mortgage at six percent. If the strong sales pattern held steady it was probable that the bank would not require that half the units be sold before they would grant the mortgage. Over seventy-five units were definitely sold by this time and there were in hand seventy-four applicants, so the outlook was optimistic.

As more and more prospective residents appeared, the task of follow-up grew to be more work than the sales and publicity forces could handle. It soon became apparent that a social director was needed: someone to keep in touch with the enrollees and to edit and send out some kind of bulletin. Mather Lippincott, Eleanor Clarke and Helen Stees were appointed to draw up a job description, while a search began for the right person. At a later meeting, Mather Lippincott announced that Joseph E. and Edith S. Platt were pursuing their application to Foulkeways and would be ideal for service in this area. The Platts were employed and made an invaluable contribution to Foulkeways for several years, both before and after they became residents.

With expanding responsibilities looming ahead, two new directors, Ella Otto and Gus Martin, were enlisted. Edward Zimmerman replaced Blanche Zimmerman on the executive board, as she was no longer able to attend the meetings.

Barclay White informed the board in October 1966 that he expected to have all living units under roof before the onset of severe weather. In a letter which was sent to "all present members of our Foulkeways family," Helen Stees wrote: "Barclay White has hundreds of men on the job. The roads are full of trucks coming and going so that just driving through to inspect is hazardous. Foundations are poured, walls are rising, and two sections of roof rafters are erected." The building went on apace all through the winter and into the spring and summer of 1967.

A group commissioned to come up with names for the thirteen building clusters went into a huddle and came up with the idea of naming them after weighty, or important, Friends who were no longer living. They cleverly put them in alphabetical order to facilitate the orientation and getting around of the future residents.

By June of 1967 all studio and one-bedroom apartments had been sold and a priority list started for them, but the two-bedroom units were not moving so well. So many of the two-bedroom apartments had been sold for single occupancy that, as early as April, the board had ruled to accept only couples, or two friends sharing one of these units, at least until the first of November. With a November opening date it was desirable that all apartments be sold and the contracts signed no later than the end of July. Publicity for the two-bedroom units was accelerated but by August 10 there were still twenty-three units unsold. There was some talk

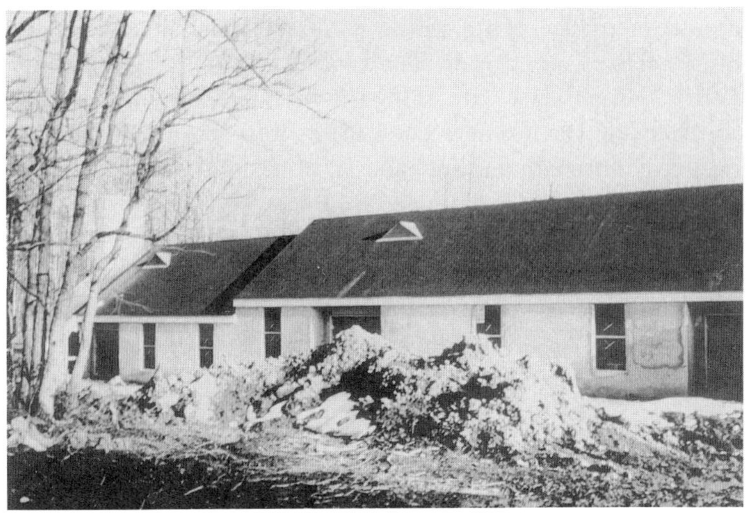

Apartment Wing Under Construction

of creating two small apartments from one large one but, fortunately, this was never done.

Allen White (who was no relation to Barclay White, Jr., the builder, and who gave up his position as business manager for the American Friends Service Committee to accept the new post) had been asked in November 1966 to be the executive director of Foulkeways. Robert Trier stayed on as administrator. Allen was to report directly to the board, with all other reports going through him. He immediately began to recruit personnel against opening day and to hold staff meetings every other week. He went to California to see how retirement communities were being run there, and he, along with those on the admissions and medical policies committees, began to formulate some rules and regulations for the efficient handling of the affairs of Foulkeways and its residents.

The criteria for getting Medicare approval for the Medical Center had to be established and met before the center could open for patients. Since there would be few convalescing residents in the early months, Foulkeways Medical Center was preparing to receive as many non-residents in the center as it could get to help defray the huge costs of running it. The costs went on, patients or no, and the outsiders would bring in much needed income. With the help of the finance committee, rates were set for the non-residents, including the non-resident spouse of a resident, as follows:

Private room with bath — $168 per week.
Private room with shared bath — $150 per week.
Semi-private room with shared bath — $100 per week.

OPENING THE DOORS

At a corporation meeting in September 1967, Barclay White set November 10 as opening day, just ten days later than his earlier projection. The vast system of volunteer committees made up of Foulkeways residents had its origin at that meeting. Future residents were asked to serve on three committees: Library, Newsletter, and Hospitality. Allen White and his staff had about six weeks to wind things up so they would be ready to go into full operation by opening day. They began to organize the sequence of the move-in dates for the residents and to notify them of their time slots.

Gwynedd Meeting received the news of the move-in with genuine delight and satisfaction, and immediately began making plans to welcome the new residents to Gwynedd Meeting and the Lower Gwynedd area. Aides from the Meeting were organized to help the newcomers in as many ways as possible.

On November 10, 1967, there was a general atmosphere of celebration among the whole multitude of those who had worked so long and hard for this day to arrive. Right on schedule, the first moving van pulled into the bleak, raw campus of Foulkeways at Gwynedd, opening what was to become the model for many subsequent Continuing Care Communities in the Delaware Valley.

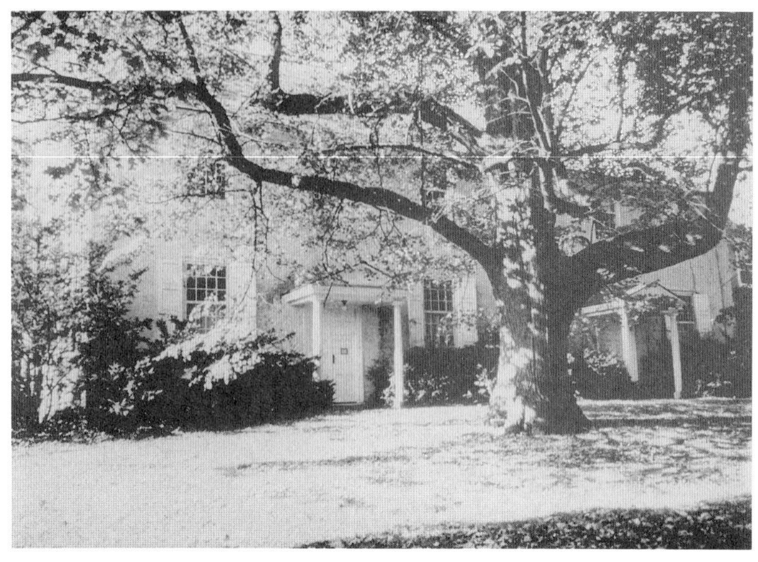

Gwynedd Friends Meeting House

Meeting was established in 1699. Present Meetinghouse was built in 1823. Addition made in 1948.

PART TWO

The Early Years

MOVING IN

On November 10, 1967, came the first settlers, strangers to each other and to the community, leaving friends and home. They came, not in covered wagons, but in moving vans loaded with furniture, heirlooms, and prized possessions — treasures piled high, often overflowing to the walks. The pioneers were frustrated; some stood and stared, others wept.

— *Otto Kronmaier,*
Foulkeways Bulletin, *November 1977*

The moving van bearing the belongings of Roger and Mariann Olden was the first to pull into the Foulkeways driveway on November 10, 1967. Mariann did not get the bouquet which had been reserved for the first resident to arrive, however, because the Oldens did not go immediately to the office. Instead, Roger directed his driver to go around to the lower level of the central building, where he could supervise the unloading of his valuable tools. Meanwhile, Herbert and Florence Thatcher arrived and went at once to the office. There Florence received the bouquet and was acclaimed the First Resident of Foulkeways.

It was a bleak picture which presented itself to those first arrivals. Building equipment and materials were still lying around, dirt was piled high in some places and little grading had been done, plus the dismal fact that the weather was drizzling and sleeting. On the third day the drizzling and sleeting turned into a full-fledged winter snowstorm, and one resident wondered aloud if perhaps Florida would not have been a better choice. Another resident lamented that the cement patios had been poured, but not the paths. Residents had to walk over the mud and snow on wooden planks. The early meals in the dining room were served on paper plates, and card tables were used until the permanent furniture was delivered.

The dreariness of the landscape was glaring even in the dark. Mary and Graham Stabler tell of arriving after dark. As the mover looked around in the dim light at the barren, treeless landscape and the plain, Quaker-like architecture, he exclaimed, "What is this place, an army barracks?" When they told him it was a retirement center, he quipped, "For retired army officers?"

The newly-assembled staff, some of the board members, and volunteers from Gwynedd Meeting and from churches of the Lansdale Ministerium were all ready and waiting for the arrival of those adventurous souls who were to be the first residents in a community offering a new way of life for older people. The plan was to move in fifteen residents a day for the first ten days.

Since the incoming residents were members of various religious persuasions, Helen Stees had asked the Lansdale Ministerium to announce to its constituent churches that

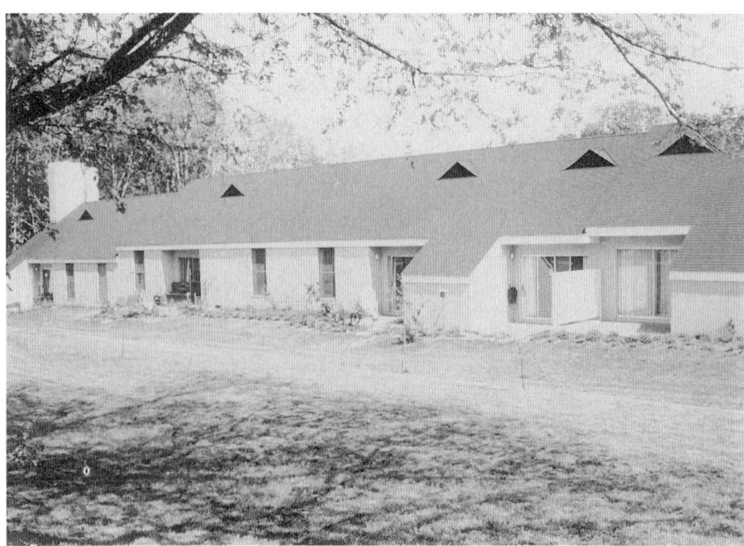

Foulkeways Apartment Wing in 1968.

volunteers to help on moving days at Foulkeways would be greatly appreciated. Some forty women from that source gave assistance over a six-week period. They were invaluable as they cheerfully helped the first residents to get settled.

To celebrate the fulfillment of the dream, the courage of the pioneer residents, and to give visibility to the new concept of aging which Foulkeways promised, Foulkeways administration and the board of directors were hosts at a reception and tea on December 17, 1967. Everybody was invited — all of Philadelphia Yearly Meeting, everyone on the priority list, the doctors from the Medical Center and their wives, the Lower Gwynedd neighbors, and friends and relatives of the residents and employees. It was a huge party and a great success. It was estimated that some five hundred persons were present. This not only made for good feelings all around, but it was an asset to the sales force in their efforts to fill the remaining two-bedroom apartments.

The board members were gratified to hear from Allen White, six weeks after opening, that the spirit of the residents was excellent in spite of all the confusion. "And confusion there is," said Allen. "The dining room is not yet working smoothly, the limousine has not arrived, the walkways are cold and windy and adequate help is hard to find." This early reference to the spirit of the residents is significant. The high expectations, the determination to make them come true, and the friendly consideration of each other which those first residents exhibited set the tone for a quality of life at Foulkeways which has never been lost. It is a rare visitor who does not remark on that felt, but intangible, dimension which seems to permeate the atmosphere of Foulkeways.

After the first big push, moving in continued steadily as apartments were finished. Final details of the building were completed by June 1968, eight months after opening. There were still 14 two-bedroom apartments unsold at that time, but by September there were only three left and by the end of the year all were occupied. Altogether there were 42

Studio apartments, 112 one-bedroom apartments and 63 two-bedroom apartments with a total population of 260 residents in the Foulkeways community at the beginning of 1969.

By that time, with all the apartments occupied and the debris hauled away, Foulkeways looked very different from the way it appeared to the first settlers when they arrived. Mud had been cleared away from the doors and the walkways had been poured. The diligent work of the residents, added to the efforts of the maintenance crew and the landscapers, had effected the transformation of a raw, ugly campus into a place of beauty and pleasure. Much remained to be done, but, already a miracle had taken place.

DECORATING FOULKEWAYS

As soon as the public areas were finished and ready to be furnished, the directors hired George Mason, a professional decorator, to be in charge. Marion Martin, Barbara Sprogell, and Helen Stees were appointed to assist him. When Helen Stees had written to future residents before Foulkeways opened to ask for contributions of books, she also said that gifts of furniture suitable for use in the public areas would be most welcome. So many things were offered that the decorating committee soon had the delicate task of deciding how to tactfully refuse what they could not use.

Many fine antiques, rugs and paintings were contributed. Also a Hammond organ for the auditorium. Four grand pianos were eventually received; two were put in the auditorium and one in each of the two parlors. Six grandfather's, or tall, clocks were given. The oldest one is probably the Bacon clock which stands in Clarke Parlor. Family legend has it that it was given to Job Bacon as a wedding gift in 1774. The large mahogany table and buffet in the small dining room were gifts, as were so many of the good pieces in the lobby of Central, the parlors in Abington House and the entrance to the Health Center. The Beaumont parlor is furnished with the antiques which Gwynedd Meeting saved from the Beaumont house. Most of the furnishings in the Clarke parlor came from William Clarke's treasured collection of English antiques.

So much of the pleasant ambience of Foulkeways is due to these beautiful pieces, some of which came from homes where they had been in the families for generations, and the good taste with which the decorating committee augmented and placed them. Lists of all these objects are in the fine arts listings (for insurance purposes) which are kept in the Foulkeways administrative offices.

Wall-to-wall carpeting and draperies were furnished for every apartment in Foulkeways. The decorating committee had the responsibility of choosing materials, colors and designs for these things as well as making decisions about wall treatments. The low-key Quaker simplicity, observed throughout, created a nice foil for the beautiful furniture and gave residents a neutral background in the apartments for the display of their personal treasures.

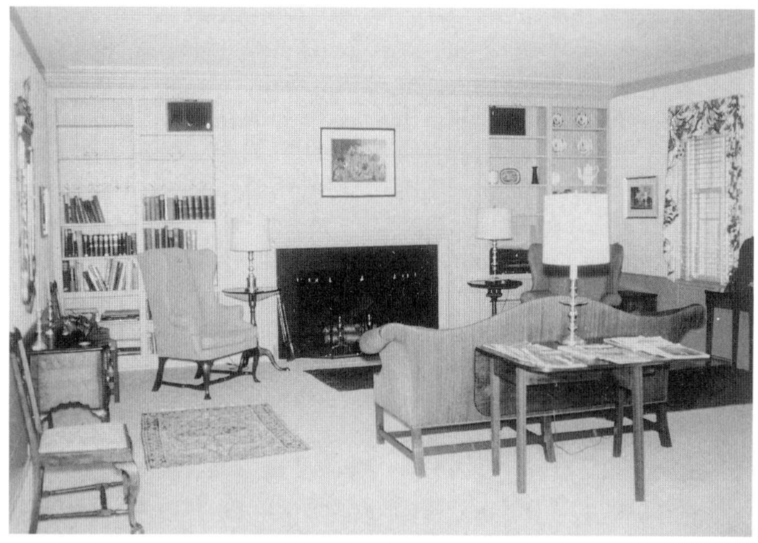

Clarke Parlor

RELIGIOUS OBSERVANCES

The first general activity in the new community was a Quaker Meeting for Worship. On November 19, just eight days after Foulkeways opened its doors, a group of Friends gathered in the auditorium for a Meeting for Worship. So runs a record kept by those early Quaker residents who assumed responsibility for the Meetings. They decided to hold a simple worship service after the manner of Friends every First-Day (Sunday) at 11 A.M., open to all who cared to attend, irrespective of denomination or religious conviction. Every week since, the Meeting has been held, with various Friends carrying out the duties involved for its proper observance. A group of from twenty-five to fifty is in attendance every Sunday. A Meeting for Worship is also held every Fifth-Day (Thursday) in the Beaumont parlor.

There is a Vesper Service held one Sunday a month in the auditorium, conducted by a clergyman from one or another of the neighboring churches or synagogues. A hymn-sing is also held one Sunday a month.

THE ADMINISTRATION

Allen White, the executive director of Foulkeways, had several assistants, or administrators, during the ten and one-half years of his tenure in that position. Robert Trier stayed on as the administrator until April 1970, when he resigned to run a Holiday Inn in the local area. He was succeeded by D. Martin Trueblood. Martin left in December 1974 to become an executive of Pine Run, a new retirement community in Doylestown, Pennsylvania. Richard Bansen succeeded Martin and held the position until after Allen retired, during which time Richard became licensed in Pennsylvania as a nursing home administrator. Allen White had been licensed in April 1972.

The skill, sensitivity and patience with which Allen White set the pattern for the future of Foulkeways was outstanding and rewarding. Armed with the knowledge of the high hopes which the founders held for their dream plus his own common sense and good judgment, he succeeded in bringing the chaos of the early days into a loving, creative, and fulfilling community.

Nancy Coppock joined the staff in 1971 as administrative assistant. That title covered anything which needed to be done and which no one else had the time to do. In the early days admissions were handled by the executive director and the administrator in a rather informal way. As word spread of the success of this breakthrough into a new way of living for the aging, increasing numbers of people came seeking admittance. More precise criteria for their acceptance had to be established. For that purpose an admissions committee was appointed from among the directors, and Nancy Coppock became the admissions coordinator and, later, the director of admissions.

Foulkeways was very fortunate in having Nancy Coppock (later Nancy Gold) as the director of admissions. In that position she has had a substantial influence on the character and climate of the whole community. She must be able to maintain a welcoming atmosphere while at the same time keep a discerning mind. That she is successful in both areas is reflected in the excellent quality of life which has been created by those which she, along with Douglas Tweddale and Patricia Miller, has recommended to the admissions committee for acceptance as residents at Foulkeways.

A priority list was started for the studio and one-bedroom units even before Foulkeways was occupied. In the early years the wait for these apartments could be from three to five years — often longer — while the wait for a two-bedroom unit was somewhat shorter. As more couples began to apply, the pattern shifted and after a few years the situation was reversed. The greater demand for the larger units continued to increase the waiting time for them.

The priority list is the only fair method of accepting applicants in an orderly fashion. It has always been scrupulously kept. No preferences are ever shown for anyone and acceptance is open to everyone on the same basis regardless of race, creed or ethnic background, with one exception. When Abington House was built, an agreement was worked out between Foulkeways and the Abington Quarter over the money which Abington Quarter advanced for the building. This agreement reserved ten priority slots at Foulkeways, in perpetuity, for members of Abington Quarter who might need a time and/or money boost. These people must still qualify for admittance in every other way, such as health and compatibility.

In September 1968 there were 23 people on the priority list. This increased to 350 by October 1970 and in February 1973 there were more than 700 on the list, even though many prospects were referred to Kendal at Longwood in Kennett Square, Pennsylvania, and to Medford Leas in New Jersey, both Quaker communities modeled after Foulkeways.

Important as the health and financial situation of an incoming resident are, the admissions director and those on the admissions committee must have a sixth sense to determine how well the applicant will fit into the life of the community. To accept a person who does not exhibit the traits which contribute to the congenial life at Foulkeways does neither that person nor Foulkeways any favor.

To help both parties in making the judgment for or against admission, the applicant must spend at least twenty-four hours on the campus, have a meal with the social worker and the director of admissions, separately, and have contact with as many residents as can be arranged. A complete tour of the facility is also conducted. Not too many mistakes are made in the process of selection, as is shown by the very few who have left Foulkeways, either of their own volition or who were gently asked to leave. A board member observed that if, perchance, there is any question as to how a new-comer is fitting in, "we begin, imperceptibly, to re-create him in our own image."

When asked why he had chosen Foulkeways, one new resident answered, "Well — I visited several retirement communities before I made up my mind, and I always checked out the parking lots. Foulkeways didn't have too many Cadillacs or Lincoln Continentals sitting around, but the cars they had were in good condition and clean. That told me what I wanted to know." Be that as it may, the Admissions Department is impressed with the number of times prospective residents mention the special spirit of Foulkeways. When new residents are asked what most attracted them to Foulkeways, their spontaneous response is almost always, "The beautiful grounds," followed quickly by, "and the friendliness of the people."

Exclusive of the administrative and health delivery staffs, Foulkeways employs over two hundred workers with a full-time equivalency of ninety-three. It is successful in retaining them. The average length of service, not counting the part-time dining room help, is six years. Many stay for fifteen to twenty years, some longer, which speaks well for the prevailing hiring and supervising policies. The generous benefits, including pensions, tax-sheltered annuity provisions, and personnel policies which Foulkeways offers are also attractive to employees. Moreover, the successful retention rate is a reflection of the pleasant surroundings and the disposition and cooperation of the residents. The rapport between administration, residents and employees is apparent to any casual observer and is an important ingredient in life at Foulkeways.

During the first four years, three directors of maintenance came and went although one of them, Ray Riday, died after only ten months on the job. Clarence Ashford took the position in October 1971 and successfully managed things until he retired eight years later.

No one worked harder during those arduous months of moving in and getting work schedules organized than the maintenance department, especially the director. The interruptions were constant; whenever anything wouldn't work or help was needed in any direction, the immediate response was, "Call maintenance. Call maintenance. Call maintenance." Small wonder the first three men did not last very long.

The spacious, beautifully-landscaped grounds, always now referred to as the campus, are one of Foulkeways' most treasured assets. The upkeep of the campus was supervised for several years by the landscapers who had designed it. Later it came under the management of maintenance, with a certified landscape gardener in charge.

Housekeeping is a separate department, though closely related to maintenance. It is responsible for all the public areas, including the Health Center and Abington House, as well as all the apartments.

When Foulkeways was being planned, it was thought that all residents would take three meals a day in the dining room. In fact, the original plans did not even include individual kitchens — only a hot plate where a resident could make a cup of tea or heat a bowl of soup. This had to be changed when the bank would not lend mortgage money for building unless there were kitchens. "What if your project fails?" they asked. "We've got to have something we can rent if that should ever happen." As the residents settled in, few of them went to the dining room for breakfast and lunch. They were required, though, to have dinner in the dining room for two reasons: this assured that the resident would have at least one balanced meal a day, and it would help administration to have some idea of the general health of the individuals.

A cafeteria became available for employees after February 1968. Not until January 1978 was it also open to residents, and this only for dinner, when there were fewer employees around. Some of the male residents had pushed for this privilege since they were not required to wear ties and jackets there as in the dining room.

THE MEDICAL CENTER

The grounds may be beautiful, the apartments comfortable, and the company congenial but the central attraction at Foulkeways is its contract for life care. All of the features of Foulkeways were planned and built to contribute to an active, creative and satisfying way of life for aging residents but the concept of life care, or continuing care as it came to be called, was the magnet which drew applicants. The Foulkeways contract guaranteed that all the medical and nursing needs of its residents, with the exception of eye glasses and dental work, would be met and paid for by Foulkeways. What a blessing to the aging and to their adult children who felt responsible for their parents' well-being.

When Foulkeways opened there were thirty rooms in the Medical Center, most of them containing two beds and very few with private baths. State approval had not been granted by opening day, nor had it been certified by Medicare. By March 1968, however, Allen White announced to the board that the Medical Center had received the highest rating possible on Medicare inspection.

The Lansdale Clinic agreed to be responsible for the delivery of medical services, with Paul L. Bradford, M.D. in charge. Sybella Sultzback, R.N. was Director of Nursing Services. The set-up was quite different in the beginning from what it evolved into later. There was no ward secretary, no social worker, no physical therapist and no pharmacy on the premises when the Medical Center opened. Nevertheless, by June 1968 there were nine residents and ten non-residents there. By February 1969 there were thirty patients in the Medical Center, ten of them non-residents.

It took awhile before the Medical Center was running smoothly, but it was finally accomplished. Mrs. Sultzback, the original director of nursing services, resigned and was replaced by Gertrude Teas, R.N. in February 1969, who was herself replaced in May 1970 by Virginia Dyer, R.N. Medicare required that there be a social worker, at the least, as a consultant. Robert Jacoby, M.S.S. was engaged for this position in September 1970. By March 1971 physical therapy was provided on a limited basis and a pharmacy with a licensed pharmacist was opened in November 1971.

There had been dissatisfaction with arrangements in the Medical Center for several months when the Foulkeways board began to think about enlarging the facilities. In September 1972 the directors appointed a committee to explore the problems and possibilities of expanding. A report of that committee includes:

> We believe that any long range solution to the Medical Center problems does involve expansion so that (a) permanent Medical Center residents who desire them may have single rooms and (b) disturbed, confused, but ambulatory residents may be cared for in a group setting which is suitable for them and less disturbing for others.

Architects from the firm of Ewing, Cole, Erdman & Eubank presented drawings for the proposed addition in June 1973. Barclay White, Jr. was selected as the builder. As usual, funding became a key issue. Richard Willis, chairman of the finance committee of the board, stated in his report that "there is reason to believe that the Residents' Association would be willing to undertake a substantial fund-raising program." The Board agreed that if the residents could raise as much as $300,000, the directors would be able to provide the balance and the work could go forward. With their usual enthusiasm, a small committee appointed by the FRA accepted the challenge and raised the money. The board set up a Foulkeways building fund to receive the contributions. The money was deposited and separately invested on a short-term basis for maximum income and used only for the Medical Center additions and improvements.

Ground-breaking for the addition was in September 1974 and dedication services were held the following May. The new wings were called Owen and Lloyd, both named for prominent seventeenth century Quaker physicians. The original wing, now called Gwynedd House, with thirty (expandable to thirty-two) beds — all with private toilets and basins — was designed for convalescing residents and for those with acute illnesses. Owen, with eighteen private rooms with baths, was for those who were there on a permanent basis, and Lloyd, with fourteen beds, was for the mentally impaired. Each wing had its own sunny, attractively-furnished lounge. There was a pleasant patio off the Lloyd lounge with the added attraction of waist-high flower beds where infirm residents could work in the soil at a comfortable level.

Since the addition of Abington House and the two new wings of the Medical Center increased the number of residents using the Abington dining room, it, along with the Abington diet kitchen, had to be enlarged. The dining room was redecorated with picture windows on one side and an attractive mural across one end.

The ground floor underneath the Abington dining room was also put to good use. The beauty shop was moved there from the crowded office area in the central building. Offices for a dentist and a podiatrist, an activities room, an office for transportation affairs and a mail box area for Abington House were also put there.

The new wings opened on June 9, 1974. Allen White reported to the board that the morale in the re-named Health Center, and in the community, was excellent and that state and Medicare approvals were imminent. One major irritation in the original wing was that the windows could never be opened. A special gift made it possible to install new windows while the other construction was going on. The new windows and individual temperature controls contributed greatly to the comfort and satisfaction of the Health Center residents.

Dr. Leland Green from the Lansdale Clinic had replaced Dr. Bradford as Foulkeways medical director in 1973. The Lansdale Clinic had given faithful service to Foulkeways from the time it opened until September 1975, when it asked to be relieved of that responsibility. James C. Alden, M.D. of Gwynedd Valley agreed to serve as medical director, releasing Dr. Green.

Patricia H. Miller, B.S., was hired as a full-time social worker in the spring of 1975 to replace Ann VanGobbes, who had been working on a part-time basis. Pat received her M.S.S. in 1979 fulfilling the Medicare requirement that there be a full-time social worker with a master's degree on the staff of the Health Center. L. Jane Kummerer, R.N., M.S.N., came to Foulkeways as the director of nursing in the fall of 1975. She was certified by the Commonwealth of Pennsylvania as a nurse practitioner, which qualified her to do routine physical examinations and prescribe simple medications. Dr. Alden and Jane Kummerer instituted an annual medical check-up of all residents with Jane doing the physicals. In addition, she and Pat Miller offered frequent seminars on health matters for the whole community.

Rose Marie Jones, R.N., who had been on the nursing staff of Foulkeways since 1971, became assistant director of nursing services, and took charge of in-service education in 1975. Elizabeth (Betty) Cash continued at the post of resident care nurse which she had so ably filled since Foulkeways was a fledgling two-week old community. Services of a dentist, Dr. Hobart Moyer and a podiatrist, Dr. Jeffry Wachtel, were made available to all the residents of the community as well as to those in the Health Center. The physical therapist continued to come in on a part-time basis and an occupational therapist was on call.

In the summer of 1973 a group of outside volunteers was organized to come in over the lunch and dinner hours to help pass out trays and to assist those who needed help in feeding themselves. They began this work before all the changes and improvements were made in the Health Center, and continued for five years throughout the building and moving upheavals. After everything had quieted down and the Health Center was running smoothly there seemed little need for their services, so the group was disbanded.

With the hope that it would help to keep the newly-won satisfaction with the Health Center at its current high level Judge Albert Maris, president of the FRA, proposed that a Health Center Advisory Council be set up to serve as a liaison between the residents, the administration and the Health Center staff. The council would consist of the executive director of Foulkeways, the director of nursing services, the social worker, the president of the FRA, an appointed resident and an outside person. The first meeting of this group was held on September 22, 1975 and it met monthly thereafter.

An unexpected fringe benefit resulted from the pur-

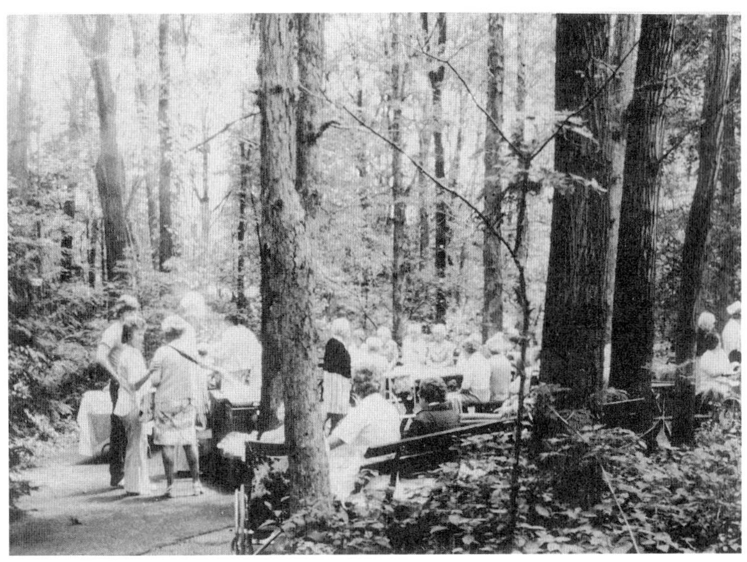

First Picnic in Abington Woods, July, 1976

chase of the wooded area when Abington House was being planned. A fairly large area in the woods was cleared of underbrush, black-topped and made accessible to wheelchairs. Picnic tables and benches were put there and a barbecue grill installed. The Health Center celebrated the Bicentennial of the United States by initiating the picnic area with a cook-out in July 1976.

THE RESIDENTS' ASSOCIATION

During that first year at Foulkeways the residents held town meetings to discuss and implement their many concerns and interests. There were so many challenging things to do, so many trivial, yet frustrating, details which needed attention, that the days were not long enough to get it all done. Yet they fell to with contagious enthusiasm to create the kind of environment and lifestyle which they had anticipated when they signed up to come to Foulkeways.

Although Quakers made up only thirty-five percent of the initial population of Foulkeways, their influence was soon felt. Committees are the backbone and mainstay of Quaker Meetings, so, in less than two months after opening day, seven standing committees had been appointed. They were: Entertainment, Flower Arrangements, Hostess, Library, Room Assignments, Special Interests, and Teas. By the time of the Fifth Anniversary in 1972 there were already eighteen active committees and more than twice that many by the end of ten years.

The nucleus of a library committee had been formed back in September 1967, when the Board was deluged with contributions in response to a letter mailed to prospective residents asking for books. Since the Foulkeways library at that time consisted of only the bookshelves which are in the lounge of the central building, decisions about which books could be used had to be made. A newsletter committee also had its origin at that September meeting of the board. Consequently, it was in position to get out the first *Foulkeways Bulletin* in January 1968. At that early date there was no residents' fund, so Administration agreed to pay Sue McMullen, Robert Trier's secretary, $300 per year to do the typing on her own time. The last issue of *Foulkeways News*, which Joe and Edith Platt had compiled and sent to all those on the priority list since October 1966, appeared in December 1967.

In order to have a framework for their activities, the residents held an organizational meeting in October 1968 to establish a residents' association. Temporary officers were named and a nominating committee appointed, as was an ad hoc group to draw up a constitution and bylaws. On December 4, 1968, the first officers and directors of the Foulkeways Residents' Association (FRA) were elected, with Charles Cook as the first president. Every resident was automatically a member of the association.

The FRA became the heartbeat of Foulkeways. The many committees which ensued were the arteries, going out into every facet of community life, giving comfort, entertainment, and education as well as opportunities for service. The interaction between the committees and the residents fostered and carried forward the feelings of fellowship and goodwill which had begun during the hectic moving-in days when they had all helped each other so much.

Problems of money and budgets must always come to the fore in any organization and the FRA was no exception. A tentative budget for the coming year was for $65 and dues were set at $1 per year. The first budget of $65 increased year by year so that, at the end of five years, the FRA treasury balance was $1,056 and after ten years it was $5,078. Where did the money, other than the yearly dues of $1 per person, come from?

From the very beginning, Foulkeways had an art gallery in the hallway of the central building. Artists were invited to hang their work on the long walls for one month at a time. When paintings were sold, the FRA collected a small percentage of the price. Profits from the gift shop were usually given to the Foulkeways Assistance Fund which was started in 1972, but money from the gift shop could also be used for the entertainment committee if necessary. A craft fair became an annual event and brought in some cash, since the FRA also took a small commission on the sales.

The big source of FRA income eventually came from the barn sales. By the summer of 1973, leftover and unwanted possessions of residents, past and present, began to clog the storage spaces. Allen White asked Nancy Coppock to hold a flea market to get rid of some of them. Thus began the lucrative business of the barn sales, which the FRA took over. A room was cleared out in the barn and made available to the barn sales committee.

In the beginning, the sales were open only to residents, employees, and their families. Sales were held on Wednesday mornings once a month during the summer. The sales for the first summer came to $1,613. This was a boon for the FRA, which began to have sufficient funds, not only for all its commitments, but for special things for Foulkeways from time to time. In 1976, for instance, the proceeds from the barn sales went toward a new bus.

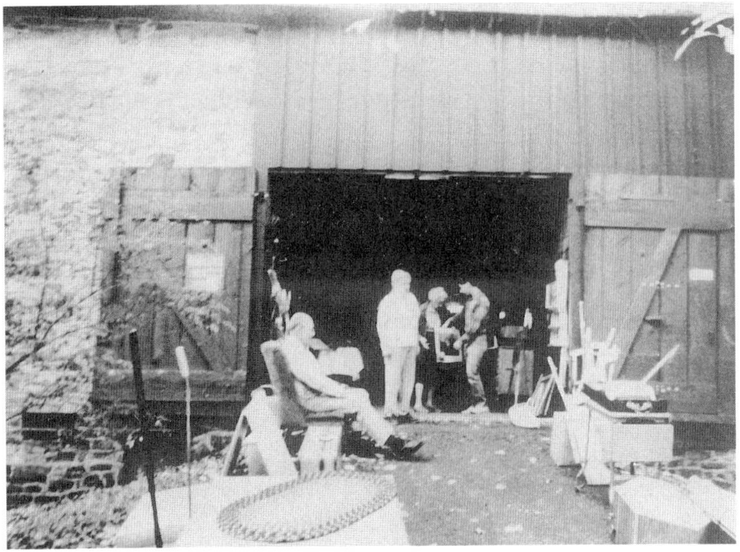

Barn Sale Day

Residents were delighted to discover, after the commotion of moving had subsided a bit, how great the advantage was of being able to board the Foulkeways bus and be driven to shopping malls, the railroad station, or even to Philadelphia and New York to attend concerts, plays, museums, and other cultural activities. The committee responsible for this also planned short trips from time to time.

Those who were not able to take advantage of outside activities had interesting things available right at home. On Monday evenings there were programs on current events and on Tuesday evenings a cultural program was presented which usually consisted of a musical program or a travelogue. Book reviews were given once a month on Saturday mornings. First-rate movies in the auditorium were a regular feature on Saturday evenings. There were also many small groups with various interests and activities.

Nicely appointed teas became the traditional way to mark special events, to greet a new official, or to say goodbye to a departing one. Teas are given each fall to honor new residents; morning coffees are held to recognize anniversary years of service of employees. The tea committee has oversight of these festive affairs. The flower committee takes care of arranging the flowers, not only for parties, but twice a week they make arrangements of fresh flowers for all the public areas.

During the first year of living at Foulkeways some customs developed which became a part of the fabric of life there. These included the tradition that there should be no door-to-door solicitations, no laundry to be hung on the patios, a dress code for the dining room, and no tipping. Since there was to be no tipping, collections would be taken in June and December for vacation and Christmas gifts to the employees. A public charitable drive, lasting for one month, was also planned for each year.

It is interesting to note that in the minutes of the FRA, until sometime in 1971, no one is called simply by his or her first name. It is always Mr., Mrs., or Miss. By the end of 1972, those titles had disappeared. The initial reserve and formality had worn off; Foulkeways had become a loving, interacting and personalized community.

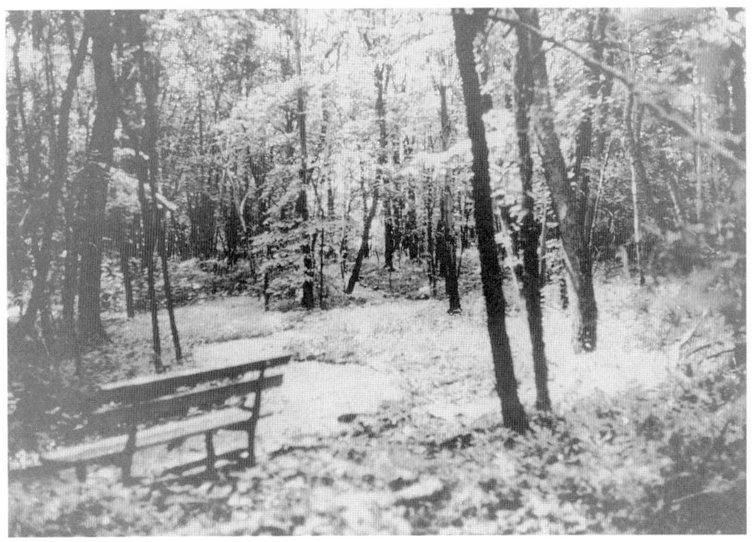

Path through the Woods

There are around four miles of walking paths at Foulkeways.

LANDSCAPING

Landscaping began as soon as the ground could be worked in the spring of 1968. Ruth Carter and Harvey Valentine, local landscape architects, along with Charles Hallowell as consultant, and the Foulkeways maintenance supervisor, Ray Riday, together with his crew, began to beautify the land surrounding the buildings.

Plantings were put in around the two entrances, and around the directional signs as they were put in place. Residents were encouraged, and received assistance as needed, to create flower beds within a three-foot limit of their patios. These became a source of great pride and pleasure and contributed immensely to the beauty of the campus. Small garden plots were laid out below the post office for any resident who wanted to have one. Over six thousand spring flowering bulbs, mostly daffodils, were planted throughout the wooded areas and around the campus. Gordon H. Ward who, along with his wife Margaret, moved into the Roeger house in 1972, wrote a forty-page *Gardening Handbook* for the FRA in 1983.

Since Foulkeways had been built on farmland, there were no trees around the buildings. The planting of trees and shrubbery was a major part of the early landscaping. Many trees were donated. Evergreen and pin oak trees from the Stees property in Kulpsville arrived and the Zimmermans contributed several young oaks from their farm in Blue Bell. Some memorial trees were also planted, though not designated as such because administration thought it might be depressing to aging residents to be surrounded by "memorial" trees. The only acknowledged memorial tree was planted in memory of Ruth Carter when she died in 1974. Ruth, who was too young to die, had given so generously of her time and talent to Foulkeways, it seemed right to honor her in this way. It helped to ease the residents' pain over her death. Trees and bushes already on the fringes of the property lines were encouraged so that neighboring houses were scarcely visible from Foulkeways.

In spacing the buildings out on the farmland, advantage had been taken of the southward slope of the fields to give a feeling of openness. Care was taken to see that each apartment would look out on beauty. The layout which made it necessary for a resident to go outside in order to get from one place to another was deliberate, thus ensuring that each person would get at least a minimum of exercise and fresh air daily.

The importance of exercise for older citizens was taken into account in the planning and landscaping of Foulkeways. Walking trails were marked out on the campus almost immediately. An excerpt from the minutes of the board shortly after Foulkeways was opened reads:

> The Board approved with proceeding to build the first section of an exercise path beginning on the Main entrance road, extending around the [west side of the buildings] ... through the woods and back to the road; then crossing the road and extending on the westerly side of [Perimeter Road] through woodland and across the entrance to the various parking lots to the access road to the Central Building. This will be built ... at a cost of $2,800.

This path, which affords so much beauty, exercise, and pleasure to the walkers, and which was built so soon after Foulkeways was occupied, is symbolic of the values the board held throughout their planning and building of Foulkeways. As more walking paths were constructed, some of the male residents saw the need for benches. They obtained kits and made many sturdy, attractive benches in the workshop, which is on the lower level of the central building. These were soon spotted along the paths and in other appropriate places where they give pleasure and comfort to everyone.

ABINGTON HOUSE

The hard-working board members were not allowed the luxury of resting on their laurels just because Foulkeways had been built and occupied. During the months of building it may have appeared that the board had forgotten the early plans of the Beaumont committee to have an intermediate stage of living which Abington House now affords. Not so. It simply had to take its turn in the scheme of things.

As mentioned earlier, in its response to the first report of the Beaumont committee in March 1959, Gwynedd Meeting had given permission for the committee to look into the possibilities of cooperating with the Abington Quarter Home Committee which had oversight of the Abington Friends Home in Norristown. Gwynedd Meeting knew that the antiquated buildings in Norristown needed more repairs and changes than seemed feasible or economical; the Beaumont committee had stated that its mission was to meet the needs of all stages of aging. Why not work together toward a common goal?

A committee consisting of Norman Winde, Dorothy Cooper, Harry Sprogell, Richard Willis and Allen White was appointed to open talks with the Abington Home committee in the summer of 1967. In May 1968, Mather Lippincott, architect, gave the board a detailed report on how a wing could be added to the Medical Center. The wing would be called Abington House. There would be sixteen rooms with private baths on each of two floors, making a total of thirty-two rooms. The main entrance would be on the ground level, facing the open meadow and the small woods. The upper level would open right into the back entrance to the Medical Center so that all the facilities of the Medical Center would be handy to the residents of Abington House.

In November 1968 the board gave instructions to Mather Lippincott, architect, and Barclay White, Jr., builder, to proceed with the construction of Abington House as soon as permits could be obtained. The final cost was set at $880,000. Of this amount the Abington Home committee of Abington Quarterly Meeting promised $200,000, and the Abington Quarter promised another $200,000. Representative Meeting of the Philadelphia Yearly Meeting gave a grant of $150,000 and a no-interest loan of $100,000 was obtained from the Chandler Fund. This left $230,000 which had to be raised through bank loans and other grants. The money from the sale of the property in Norristown was to go to the building fund, but no buyer was found until January 1973, over four years later. The property brought $75,670 and the contents sold for $7,600, making a total of $83,270, which was turned over to Foulkeways.

The hope was to have the new wing ready for occupancy by December 1969 but there were delays. A neighbor was concerned that the end of the proposed building came too close to the property line. Instead of going through lengthy township hearings, Foulkeways purchased three and one half-acres of woodland, which eliminated that problem. Other postponements, some due to labor problems, occurred, however, so that it was not until September 1970 that construction was finished and preparations were made for occupancy. Twenty rooms were filled immediately. Six residents came from Norristown, six from Foulkeways Medical Center and eight from the apartments. Full occupancy of the thirty-two rooms was expected by March 1971.

Abington House is described as a personal care facility with some custodial care. To be accepted at Foulkeways, residents must be ambulatory and must be able to function independently in an apartment. When the time comes that this is no longer possible, but the person does not yet need nursing care, that person is moved to Abington House. Here there is supervision and help as needed — with baths, medications, or dressing — until it becomes necessary for the person to be moved into the nursing center. Residents in Abington House are served breakfast on a tray in their room and they may go to either the Abington House dining room, or to the main dining room for lunch and dinner (unless they must be in a wheelchair).

Shortly after Foulkeways opened, the residents themselves decided there should be no wheelchairs in the main dining room; it would be too depressing. There were some in administration who were not comfortable about this, but since most, if not all, of those who required a wheelchair lived in the Medical Center and had their meals in the Abington dining room, this never became a big issue. Residents in the Medical Center have access to all of the activities of Foulkeways and are members of the FRA.

MAINTENANCE BUILDING

All the time that Abington House was being built, the maintenance department was impatiently waiting for a building to house their equipment. By that time, all of Foulkeways' grounds had been landscaped and required more attention than had been necessary in the beginning. Since more equipment was needed for the extra work involved in the upkeep of the grounds and buildings, it became obvious that a maintenance building was sorely needed. Plans for it had been brewing for some time but, since it could not be started until after Abington House was finished, it had to wait. Work was finally begun in November 1970 in the area of the barn and post office near Meetinghouse Road, and proceeded quickly. It was finished by the following February. Further additions were made and the surrounding area was black-topped as time went on until there was adequate space to house most of the equipment, including the two Foulkeways buses.

THE BARN

There were some who thought the old Pennsylvania bank barn alongside Meetinghouse Road posed a hazard and should be taken down. Others saw it for the asset it is — an attractive old stone and frame barn which gives character to the place and provides much-needed storage space. After all the trappings pertaining to maintenance had been cleared out, it was used for the barn sales and for storing summer furniture for the residents. It was not repaired until 1978 when four steel rods were installed across the width of the building to prevent further bulging of the walls. A lintel was placed over the main double doors on the lower level, holes were patched and broken windows replaced.

The doors on the lower level opened out onto the black-topped area around the maintenance buildings, which made the lower level an ideal place to store various supplies for building and upkeep. A big door on the upper level, made wide enough originally to accommodate large loads of hay, opened onto the barn bank and the road. Trucks loaded with furniture could back right up into the opening for loading and unloading.

OTHER HOUSES

When Doris Jones, who had continued to live in the Lowry House after Edwin Jones's death in 1969, moved into Foulkeways in 1972, the board had to decide on the best use of that property. Requests had come from some people on the priority list for permission to build a cottage somewhere on the property. This would give them more space and privacy than was available in the apartments, and would also enable them to get into Foulkeways more quickly. This was considered, for there is enough land there for a cluster of cottages, but was rejected. Instead, in 1974, the Lowry house was renovated. A large apartment was created on the first floor and two guest rooms with private baths were made available on the second floor. By 1972, five years after opening, it had become apparent that guest rooms for visiting families of residents would be a most welcome addition to Foulkeways. Two more were added later when another house was bought.

The Roeger house on Meetinghouse Road, just past the original Foulkeways model units, was bought in 1972. With no changes, it remained a single residence for several years. Later it was made into two apartments for residents, and with the Lowry House and the two apartments which were made from the model unit, was named Sprogell. Harry Sprogell, who had given so very much of his wisdom, time and energy to Foulkeways, had died on New Year's Day, 1972.

THE BOARD OF DIRECTORS

In the beginning, back in 1963, there was the Foulkeways Association, consisting of from thirty to forty persons, and the Foulkeways Organization Committee composed of eight to ten persons. The Organization Committee soon came to be called the Executive Committee. The Executive Committee continued to meet in Harry Sprogell's law office in Philadelphia until September 1970. Thereafter, it met at Foulkeways. During the seven years that it met at Harry's office, he not only furnished space for the meetings, he also allowed the secretarial services of his office to be used for Foulkeways, a major contribution.

Harry Sprogell's death on January 1, 1972, was a blow to everyone connected with Foulkeways. The board tried to express its grief at its meeting three weeks later, as follows:

> The Board of Directors met ... with a profound sense of personal loss in the death of Harry Sprogell, our vice-president. Harry's sensitivity and concern for the legal as well as the personal problems of our residents was only a small part of his lasting contribution to the community. ... He gave of himself tirelessly to the planning, financing, and making a reality of the Meeting's dream.

By unanimous approval his wife, Barbara S. Sprogell, was appointed to membership on the board.

Annual meetings of the association members were held in May, first at Gwynedd Meeting and later at Foulkeways. In the planning and building years the members of the association were needed for the help they were able to give in many areas. After Foulkeways was occupied and working smoothly there was little need for the association. In April 1973 the minutes of the board report that there is no longer a legal requirement to have members of a corporation different from members of a board of directors. The alternative would be to have only a board of directors, the members of which would constitute the entire membership of the corporation.

Alan Hunt, Esq., counsel for the board, recommended that it would be to the board's advantage to dissolve the original Delaware corporation and re-incorporate in Pennsylvania under the new structure. Foulkeways was incorporated in Delaware in 1964 because of the favorable and flexible laws of that state for incorporators. By 1974 the laws in Pennsylvania had become more attractive regarding corporations, hence Alan Hunt's recommendation.

All members of the association were informed by letter of the proposal and asked to register their approval or disapproval of the action. Proxies were enclosed for those who could not come to the meeting. The change took place, effective January 7, 1974, and the name of the Pennsylvania corporation became Foulkeways at Gwynedd, without the "Inc.". Letters of appreciation, expressing the gratitude of the board for their years of service and interest, were sent to all the retiring association members. All of the officers of the Delaware corporation remained in their respective offices after the change and were re-elected on May 20, 1974.

The board of directors had never stipulated any size of that body nor the length of time a member should serve. It was self-perpetuating, except for two members which the Abington Quarter Home Committee nominated. Members were appointed as seemed appropriate and stayed on as long as they wished to serve. When the 1974 changes were taking place, some rules were established for the composition of the board. It was decided that eighteen members would make a good working size. There would be three panels of six, with six to be named each year. Maximum length of service on the board would be limited to three terms of three years each, with the exception of the president of the board. No limits were set for that office. After an absence of a year, a person became eligible to be reappointed.

Because some residents had been campaigning to have representation on the board of directors, in the fall of 1976 Alan Hunt was asked to give the matter some thought and come in with recommendations. In his report in November 1976 he recommended that there be a "modest representation" of residents on the board. They should be appointed in the usual way by the incumbent board members and they should be members of the Religious Society of Friends. At the board meeting in January 1977 Albert B. Maris and Linda C. Paton were approved and invited to serve as the first residents on the board of directors.

The desire to attract minority members as residents to Foulkeways was a recurring theme at the board meetings. In September 1974 Norman Winde reported to the board that Gwynedd Meeting had raised questions about this subject in one of its monthly meetings. Allen White reported to the board in January 1976 that:

> Foulkeways has made a special effort to ... be open to members of minority groups to become residents. ... It is now proposed that Foulkeways cooperate with Kendal to seek out someone with background and experience [in this field] to represent Foulkeways and Kendal to minority groups.

Although minority groups have always been well represented among its employees, Foulkeways has never been successful in attracting more than a few as residents, even though individual and corporate efforts have been made.

Norman Winde, who became the second president of the board in 1965 after William Clarke died, held that position for ten years. He carried a heavy load during the planning and construction years. He and Harry Sprogell had often served as an executive committee of two in the early years, in that they were called upon to make decisions of great

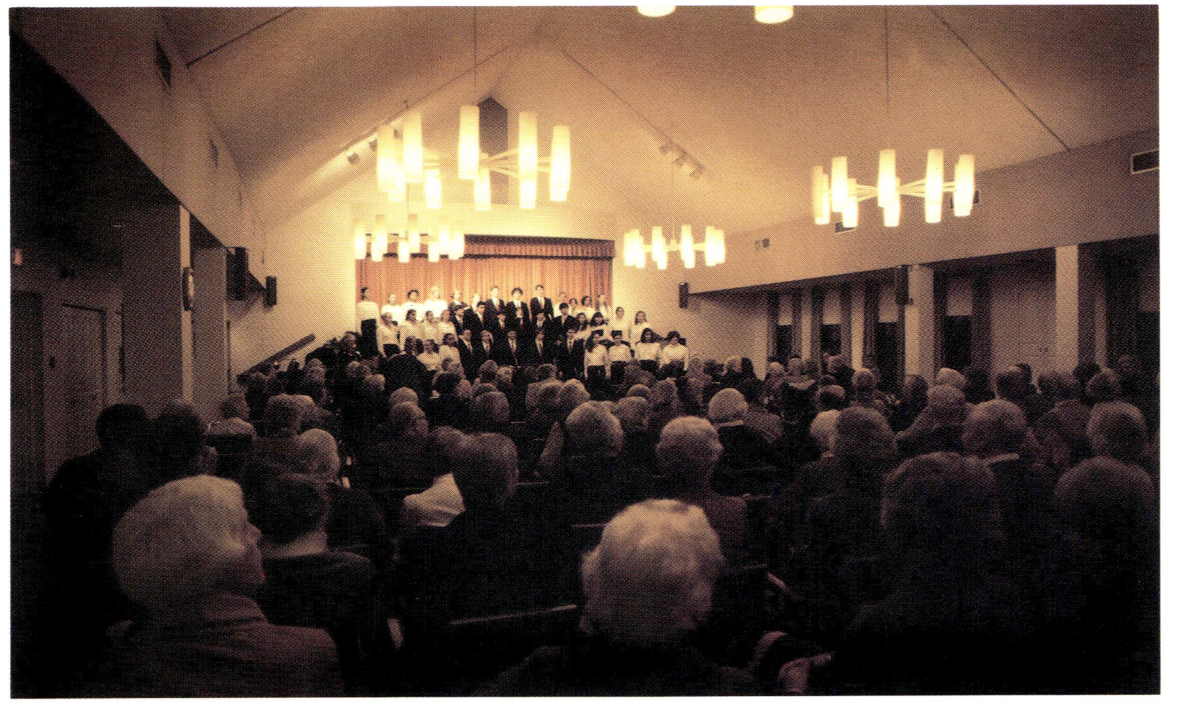

Auditorium and Multi-Purpose Room
during a concert by the Germantown Friends School Choir

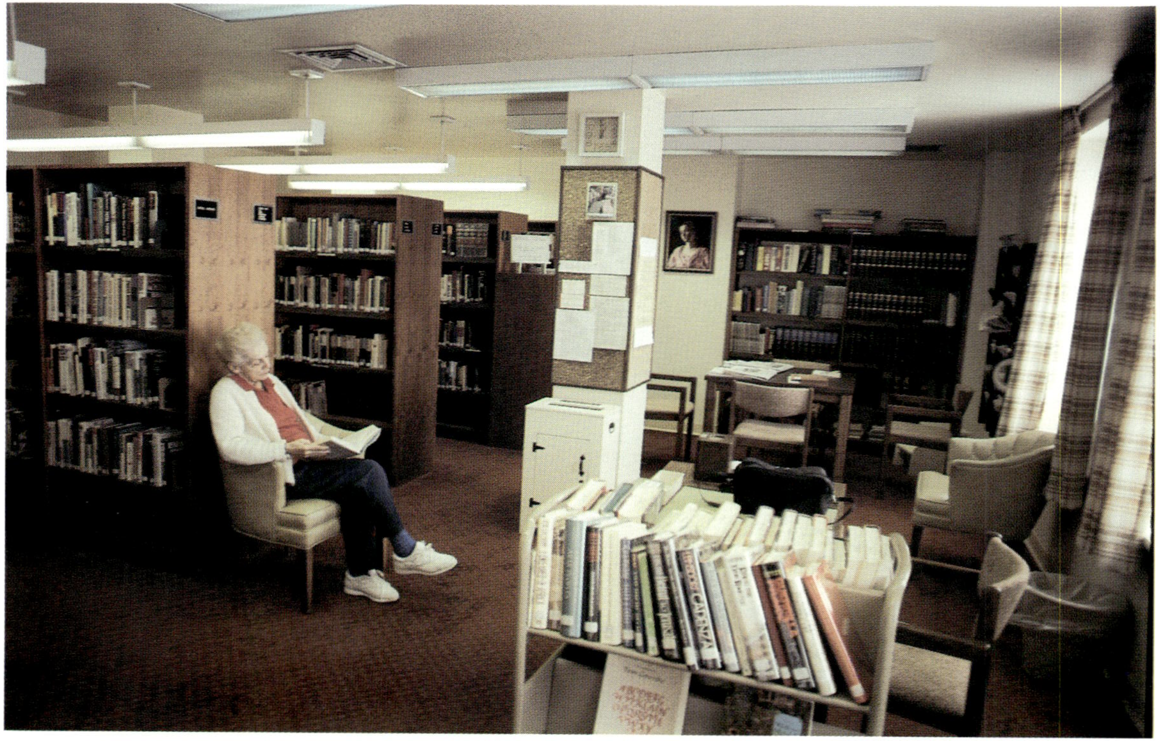

Library

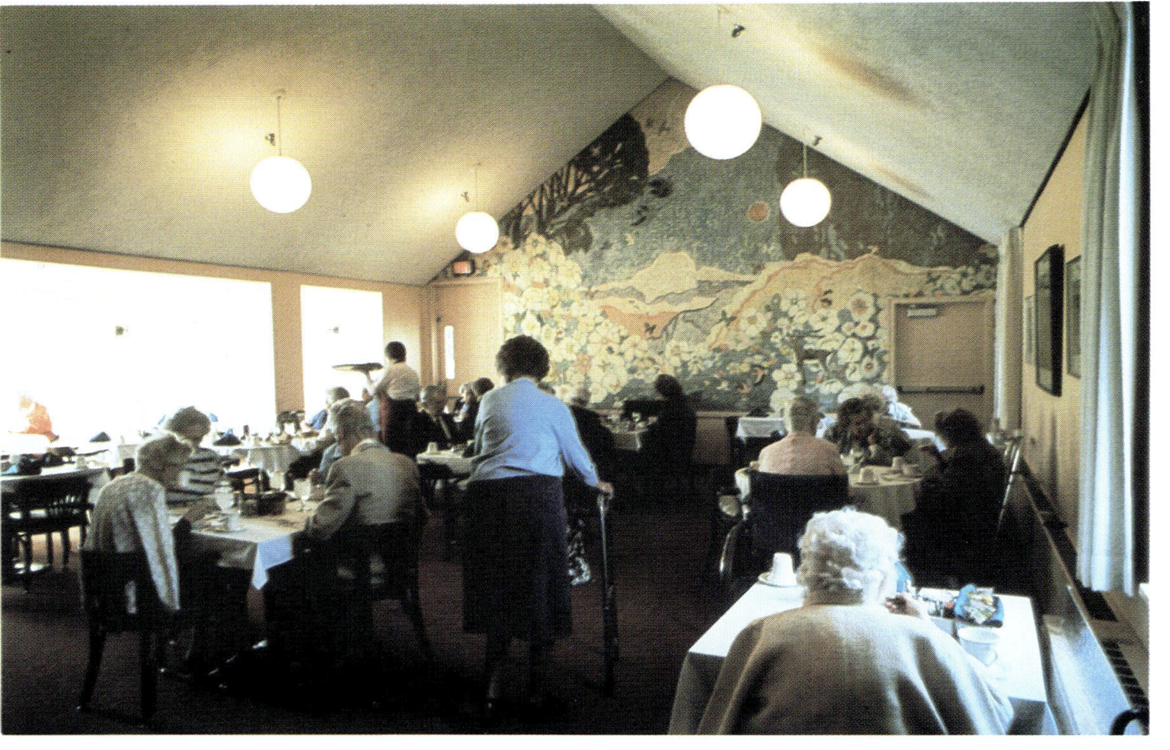

Abington Dining Room

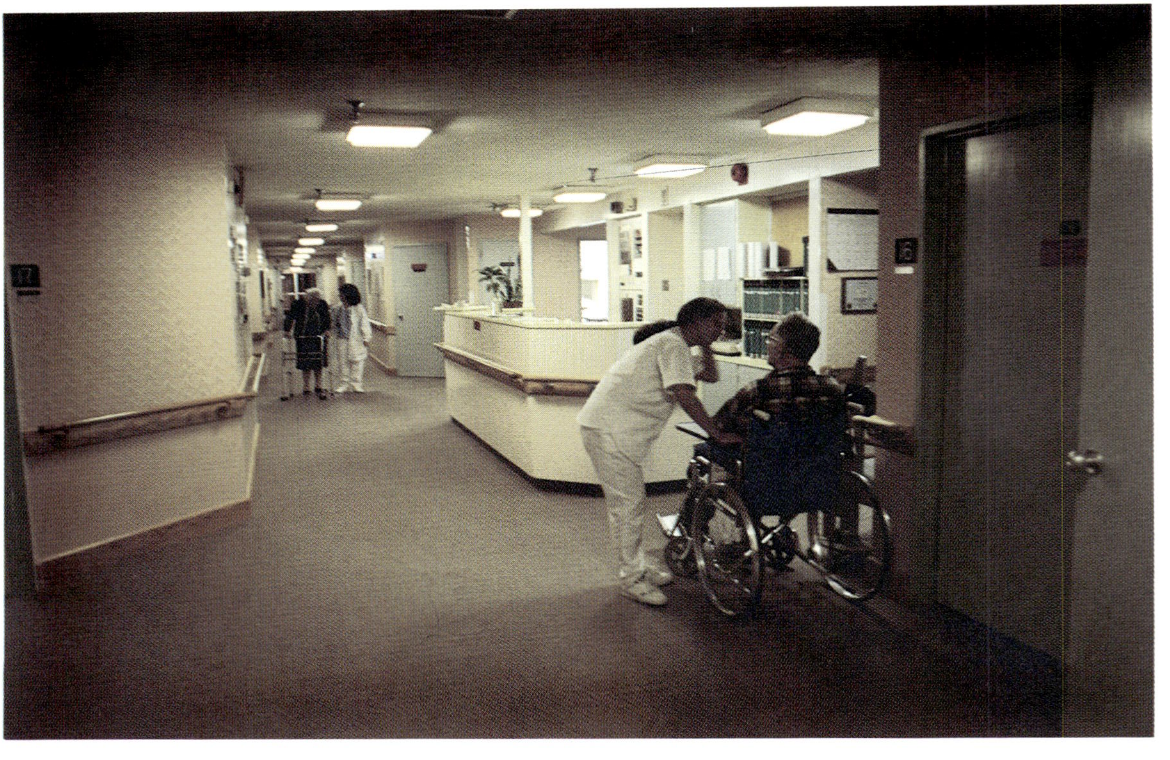

Health Center — Gwynedd House

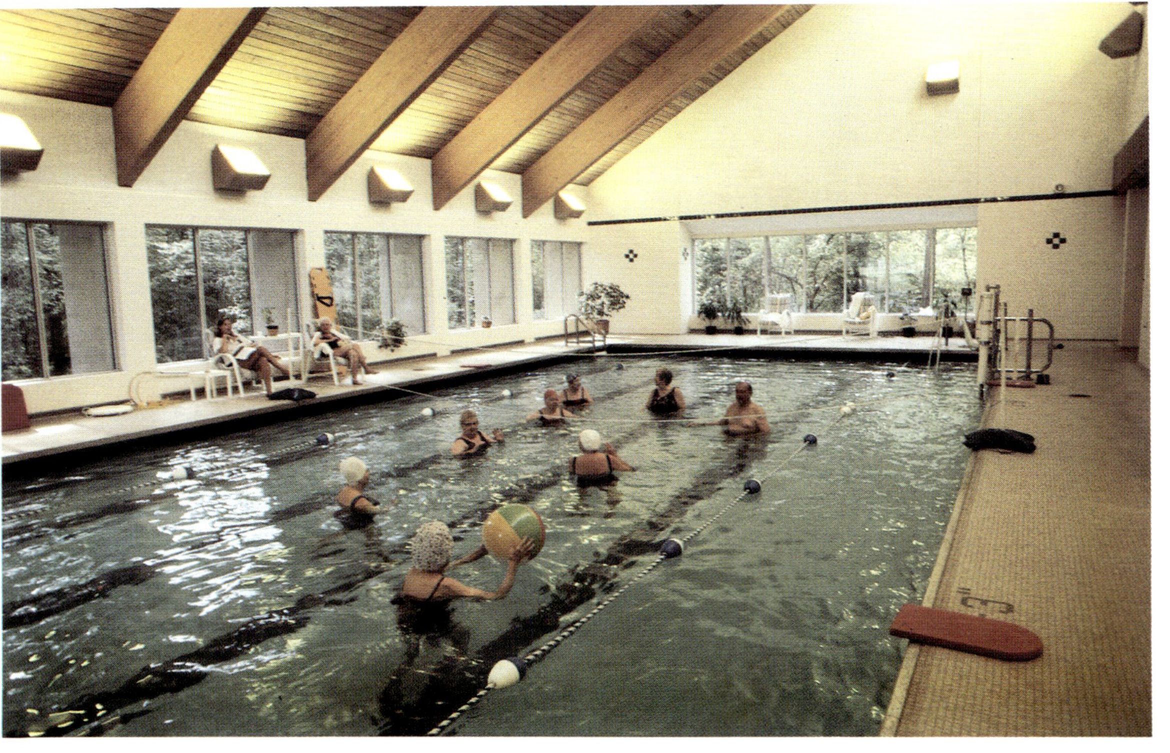

Swimming pool / volleyball game in progress

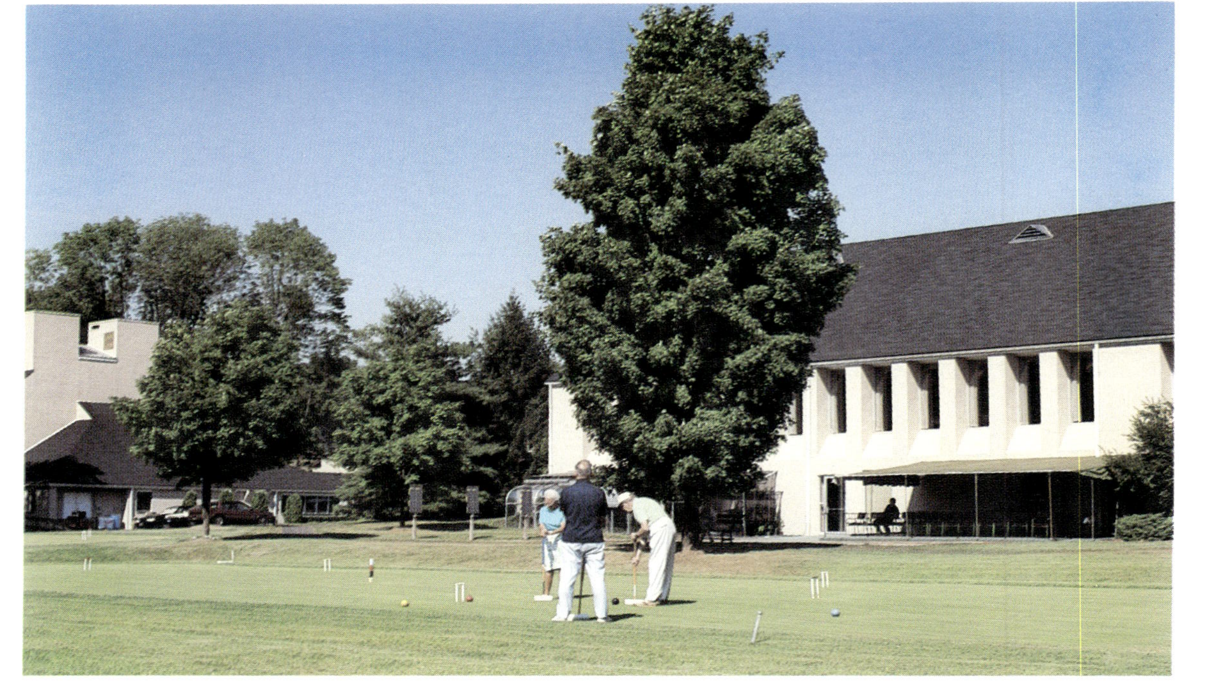

Wimbledon Court

The building on the right is the back view of Central, showing windows of dining room (left), Central lobby (center). The auditorium (not shown) is to the right. The building to the left is the Natatorium.

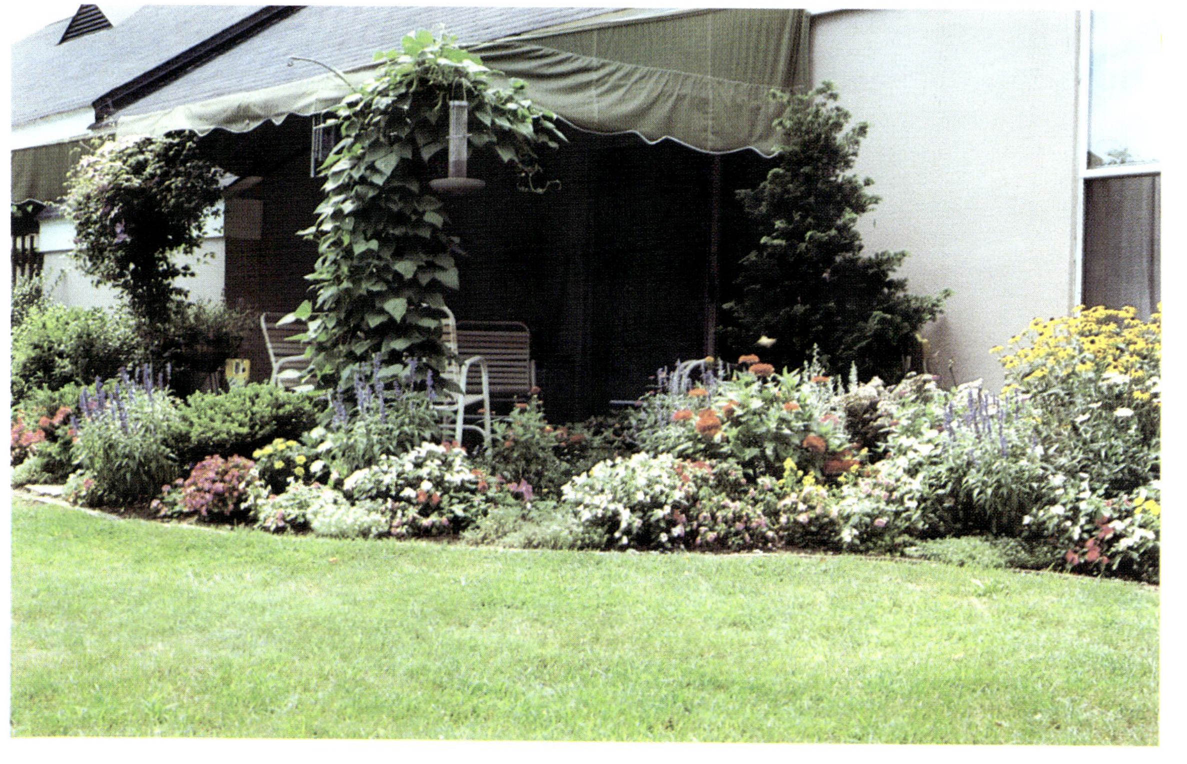

A resident's patio and flower beds.

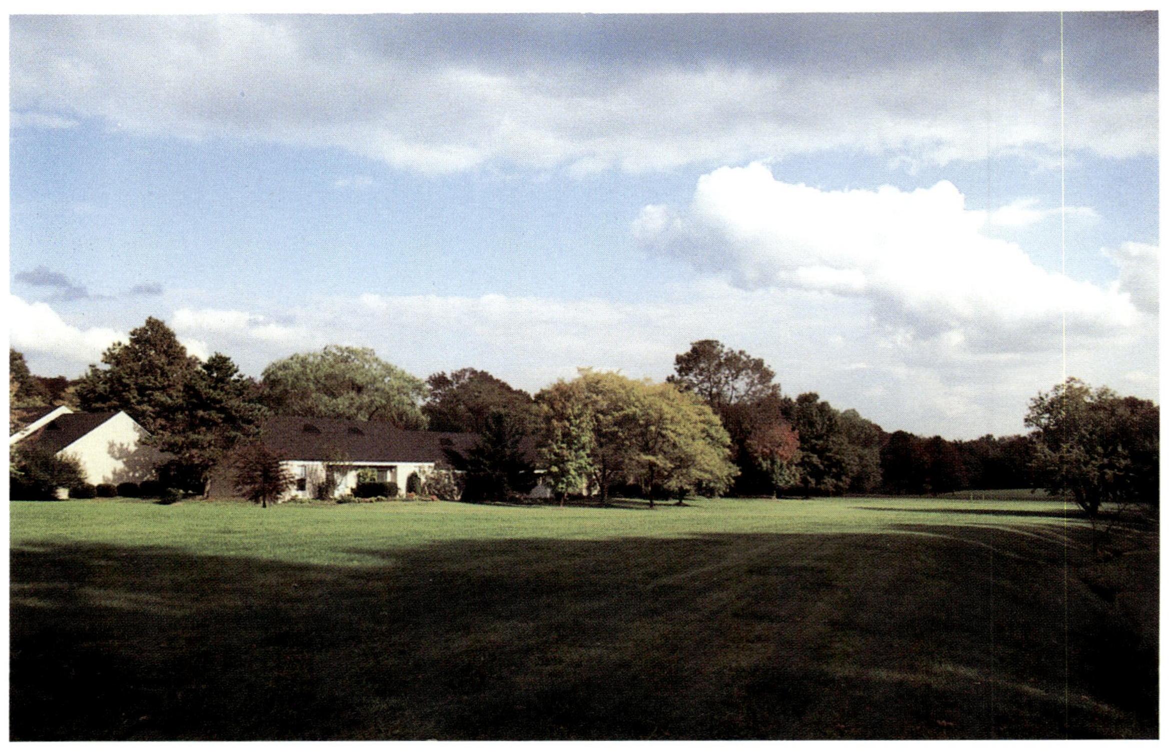

Looking south from Central across the meadow

consequence between board meetings when no one else was available. Norman Winde resigned and was designated president emeritus in May 1975. At the annual meeting of the corporation on May 27, 1975 excerpts from the minutes read:

> The Foulkeways Board wishes to minute its very real appreciation of the dedicated, wise and unstinting efforts of its retiring president, Norman H. Winde. .. [He began] his work as the second president of the Foulkeways Corporation two and one-half years before the Foulkeways Community officially opened to residents. ... His manner, his thoughtfulness and his intense concern for the well-being of the residents and the financial soundness of the project have been extra-ordinary.

Richard B. Willis, who had succeeded Thomas Elkinton as treasurer of the board, was unanimously selected to be the new president. He began his duties with the May 1975 meeting. In a letter which he sent out to the residents while he was President he stated that "the prime responsibility of the Foulkeways Board of Directors is to assure the financial integrity of the community and thereby the financial security of its residents."

It is obvious that he was constantly mindful of that responsibility. Even a cursory reading of the minutes of the board of directors shows its consistent attention to the finances of Foulkeways. This is reflected in the fact that Foulkeways has always been on a very sound financial basis. A retired banker who moved to Foulkeways stated that before he made his decision to come, he examined the financial statements of all the leading retirement facilities in the area and found that Foulkeways was in the strongest financial position of them all.

The central building which houses the Community Center, (which came to be called simply Central), is the geographical and functional center of Foulkeways. The office area in Central, which was adequate for accommodating the affairs of the board, the administration, and the residents when Foulkeways first opened, very soon began to seem crowded.

Originally, the beauty shop and the gift shop were in one room in the rear of the office area. When Abington House was built, the beauty shop was moved there and the gift shop was moved just inside the front entrance. This relocation gave the gift shop a little more room but it was still too small and it did not increase the office space at all. Nevertheless, it was not until 1977 that this was changed.

Richard Willis reported to the board in September that the executive committee had decided to proceed with enlarging the central building in order to expand the gift shop, increase the mail box area and create two new offices. This was done by pushing the front wall outward and eliminating a strip of grass which was between the building and the walk. The work was begun immediately and was finished by the end of January 1978, when the whole office area was redecorated and repainted.

As early as 1971 a committee of staff and residents met to study the lower level of Central and make recommendations for its greater usefulness. No space was added, but after some maintenance supplies there were moved to the new maintenance building, more space was available for other things. A weaving room and a branch bank were thereupon installed. An arts and crafts room was already there, as was a woodworking shop. What was originally thought of as a "Men's Clubroom" was turned into a room for table games.

An outdoor games area had been created at the rear of the ground level of Central. Later, a furnished and fitted patio, with an awning, was added for comfortable spectator participation.

Furthermore, the committee which had effected the changes in the lower level in 1971 had also recommended at that time that the auditorium be enlarged to include a permanent stage, with two dressing rooms. The original movable stage was not large enough to accommodate the kinds of programs which the entertainment committee was bringing to Foulkeways, nor was there enough seating space for the audience. However, this was not accomplished at that time for several reasons.

When Foulkeways was designed, all of the walkways were put on the outside of the buildings and the apartments for the purpose of getting the residents out in the open air as much as possible. Fresh air or no, the cold, winter blasts caused so much discomfort that in 1972 the walks immediately approaching the entrance to Central were enclosed with glass windows. This area, soon dubbed the "glass tunnel," was made possible by a grant of $8,500 from the Chace Fund. In addition slatted wooden windbreaks were gradually put up along the most vulnerable places on all other walks for the winter months.

Other improvements through the years included automatic doors at the entrances to Central, the Health Center and Abington House. Storm windows in all apartments and insulation over the ceilings of the apartments not only made for greater comfort but provided a saving in heating costs of over $10,000 the first year and each year thereafter.

The opportunity to buy the Poole property, which adjoined Foulkeways along its north eastern boundary, coincided with the desire of three or four individuals to build, at their own expense, cottages on Foulkeways land and under a Foulkeways life care contract. The individual cottage idea was rejected but the prospect of acquiring that particular property where a few more apartments could be built was appealing. Richard Willis and Allen White met with the residents to explain the proposed development and answer questions. The minutes of the board for June 1976 reflect the thinking of the directors and their plans to keep the residents informed of what was going on:

> While the Board made no determination as to the number of apartments it was willing to construct ... it was agreed that the number should remain small and that full consideration should be given to the adequacy of common facilities ... and to keep the total number in the community at a level which would not, in any way, damage what we like to think of as the "Foulkeways spirit".

The ground was purchased shortly after that meeting. The architectural firm of Ewing, Cole, Erdman, Rizzio & Cherry was engaged as architects, engineer, and planners; Barclay White, Jr. was again the board's choice as the builder. By April 1977 the plans for building seventeen apartments (one of which was a studio apartment) on the seven-acre plot had crystallized. The architecture of the buildings was similar to the design of the existing buildings, inside as well as out.

So that the new buildings would not add to the financial burden of the existing residents, the cost of the ground ($45,000) was figured in the entry fees of those who would occupy the new apartments. Future residents, whose acceptance was based strictly on their priority list position, were asked to put up half the cost of the facility of their choice when they signed up, the balance when they moved in.

When the construction committee met on July 25, 1977, the admissions director — now Nancy Coppock Gold — had commitments for each of the apartments and deposits were being received for the first half of the entry fee. In a report to the board two months later, Gus Martin, chairman of the property committee, reported that "the 7-acre project is progressing and it is hoped that it will be ready by March 1978." The names chosen, which needed to begin with "P" and "R" to continue the alphabetical run which had been used for the original apartments, were Pickett and Rowntree.

TRANSITION TO A NEW EXECUTIVE DIRECTOR

Foulkeways had not set out to build a better mousetrap, but it had not been long in existence when the world began to beat a path to its door. Often they came individually; sometimes they came by the busload. Shortly before the residents moved in it was on the route of the Lansdale Christmas Caravan, a benefit tour which visited places of interest in the area. A busload came from Riverside Church in New York. Another bus arrived bearing Friends from New Jersey who were interested in starting a similar facility, and in 1973 two busloads of representatives from the American Association of Homes for the Aging came to visit.

Word of the new retirement community in Lower Gwynedd Township spread across the Delaware Valley. Just as members of the Foulkeways organization committee went to California back in 1963 to see what had been done in the field, so interested people east of the Mississippi now came to Foulkeways.

As more and more of Allen White's time was being taken up by advice seekers, it became necessary for Foulkeways to charge a fee for his services. In 1973 Norman Winde informed the board that Allen was serving as a paid consultant in the field of retirement centers for the architectural firm of Ewing, Cole, Erdman & Eubank, as well as meeting with other groups and individuals. Consequently, many of the retirement communities in the area bear the imprint of Foulkeways in their designs and contracts. Certainly, the earlier ones do.

In 1973 Foulkeways entered into a contract with Medicon, Inc., a consulting service for retirement communities, whereby Foulkeways would be paid an agreed-upon fee for Allen White's time. Medicon later changed its name to Life Care Services, Inc., and became registered in Pennsylvania. Its mission was explained to the board in these terms:

> Life Care Services, Inc. is interested in expanding services to the aging by providing consulting services to organizations which would provide life services ... much on the order of those provided by Foulkeways. ... Any income [returned to Foulkeways from Life Services] will acknowledge the role of Foulkeways.

An agreement between Foulkeways and Life Care Services, Inc. was accepted and signed for Foulkeways by Richard Willis, president of the board, in April 1977. At that time, Life Care Services was working with five different groups; less than a year later there were nine under its care.

Allen White had been the executive director for ten years when he asked the board to look for a replacement for

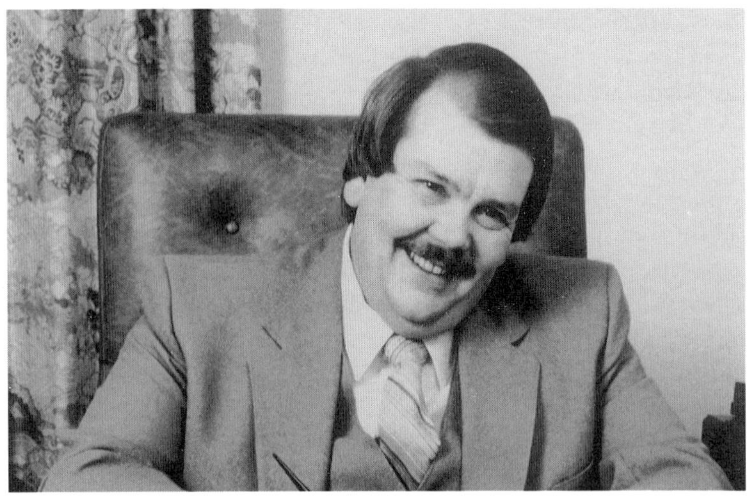

Donald L. Moon
Executive Director 1978–1990

him. He had served on the board of directors for four years before Foulkeways opened, making a total of sixteen years of continuous service to the care of the aging. In June 1977 the selection committee, chaired by Cornelia C. Schmidt, presented its choice. Donald L. Moon was unanimously approved by the board. He came from Indianapolis, Indiana, where he was pastor of the First Friends Church there. His title for the first year at Foulkeways would be associate director and his duties would begin in September 1977. On September 18, 1977, Donald and his wife, Carolyn, were introduced to the community at a reception held in the lobby of Central.

To facilitate the transition it was agreed that Allen White would stay on as executive director until March 31, 1978, at which time Donald Moon would assume all duties relating to the administration of Foulkeways, still keeping the title of associate director. Allen would continue to serve as the executive director until September 1978 and be available as a consultant until January 1, 1979.

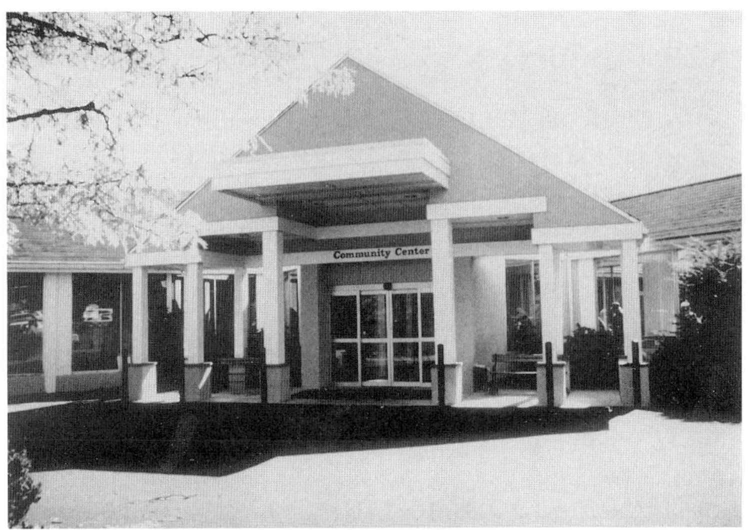

Entrance to Central

Meanwhile, the work load was increasing for Allen in Life Care Services, Inc. Since Donald Moon had assumed all the duties of executive director on April 1, 1978, the way was clear for Allen White to give up that position on the first of June instead of waiting until September. He could then give his whole attention to the consulting business, which had recently been reorganized and re-named Third Age Associates.

Allen and Ellen White were honored at a tea on June 11, 1978. The outpouring of respect and affection toward them from the residents, staff and employees was a mighty tribute to both of them. Ellen White had always been visible during Allen's tenure at Foulkeways. She and Allen had dinner in the dining room at Foulkeways several times a week in an effort to know the residents and to keep an eye and ear on what was happening in the new community. She was present at important occasions and it was she who initiated the custom of having fresh flowers, paid for by administration, in the public areas. It was also her suggestion that there be a photograph album of the residents in the lobby of Central. The photographs are a great help to new residents as they try to match names to faces in their first confusing days as residents at Foulkeways.

When Allen White assumed the duties of executive director of Foulkeways with the responsibility of launching the first continuing care community in the area, he faced a formidable challenge. The minutes of the board of directors and the FRA are a testament to his accomplishments. Along with the smooth running of the establishment, there was always, as one resident expressed it, a "hum of contentment" in the atmosphere of Foulkeways. Allen's was the steady hand and the pleasant smile during the hectic months while the character and the unique philosophy of Foulkeways was being forged, and where far-reaching policies were being instituted. He left an enduring legacy to a happy, healthy, and financially secure establishment when he handed the directorship over to Donald Moon in June 1978.

Allen White died on March 23, 1989 as he and Ellen were making arrangements to become residents of Foulkeways. At a meeting of the Board on May 22, 1989, the following minute was approved:

> The Foulkeways Board of Directors was saddened to learn of the death of Allen J. White, the first Executive Director of Foulkeways from 1967 through 1978. He successfully completed the exhausting task of start-up and was, to a large extent, responsible for the tone of Foulkeways and the esprit of the residents and staff, which continues to exist. The affection both groups had for Allen and their harmonious activity ... reflected his interest and concern for them. ... We remain grateful to Allen J. White for his strong leadership.

PART THREE

Continuing Care

THE RESIDENTS' ASSOCIATION

Donald Moon's first address to residents at the semi-annual meeting of the Residents' Association on June 15, 1978, evoked feelings of accomplishment and satisfaction among them. "Here is not a typical institution," stated Don. "Why?"

Then he listed the characteristics he saw being lived out at Foulkeways which justified his observations. They were: "(a) the caliber of the people, (b) a sense of community — a thing of the spirit, (c) a noticeable willingness to help each other, and, (d) a pervasive element of caring."

The first one, the caliber of the people, could be attributed to the quality and simplicity of Foulkeways which draws a certain kind of person to it. The other three elements are largely due to the wisdom which the administration and the board of directors demonstrated in the early days of Foulkeways when they decided against having a formal activities director. For a year or two, the board did have a committee on resident activities, which gave suggestions and help in planning their early activities, but it was laid down as the residents themselves began to take over. Out of the efforts of the residents to enrich their own lives grew the sense of community, the willingness to help each other, and the element of caring which Don Moon had recognized.

As Foulkeways entered the second decade of its existence the community continued to thrive with spontaneity and vigor. The life of the vibrant community was expressed in and through the committees of the Foulkeways Residents' Association, or the FRA as it was usually called. In 1977 there were thirty-four active committees; by 1990 there were fifty-four. Not only was the interaction among the residents important for the health of the social organism, it also supplied money for ongoing activities. By 1990 the balance in the FRA treasury was a whopping $35,448. As was said of the early Quakers in America, they set out to do good and they did well.

The FRA is managed by an executive board made up of a president, vice-president, secretary, treasurer, and six other members as well as the out-going president. All officers and members are appointed for a term of two years. The vice-president moves up to the presidency after serving two years as vice-president. There is an executive committee composed of the president, vice-president and one other member. The president, along with the board, appoints the chair of all committees; the chair then selects the committee members according to the scope of that committee. There is no limit on the terms the chairs or the committee members can serve.

The directors of the FRA meet ten times a year, with an annual meeting in January and a semi-annual meeting in June, open to all members of the association. Committee reports are given at these meetings. To make the reports manageable the committees are divided into four major categories: cultural activities, artistic expression, practical mechanics and services.

The *cultural activities* committees cover everything from planning for concerts, lectures, and slide shows in the Foulkeways auditorium to arranging for bus trips to the Academy of Music, the theater or museums in Philadelphia. Trips to other concerts and lectures in the area are arranged, as well as trips to the opera and museums in New York. This group also manages the library, and is in charge of the teas and parties at Foulkeways and all other things of a cultural nature.

Individual creativity of the residents is encouraged and augmented through the work of the *artistic expressions* committees. A large arts and crafts room accommodates various classes: painting, sketching, and ceramics — with a kiln for finishing the ceramics creations. Equipment for cutting out and sewing is also in the arts and crafts room, and there is a separate weaving room. A darkroom caters to the camera clubs and there is a well-equipped wood-working shop. Many fine pieces of furniture have come out of the wood-working shop, and beautiful objects of art have been produced by Foulkeways residents. Frequently-changed display cases on the lower level of Central allow the creations of residents to be enjoyed.

The annual Foulkeways Arts and Crafts Fair in the fall is one of the major events. It allows residents an opportunity to display their work and it furnishes a market for them. This helps not only the creator of the wares; it enables house-bound residents to buy unusual things for their own pleasure or for gifts.

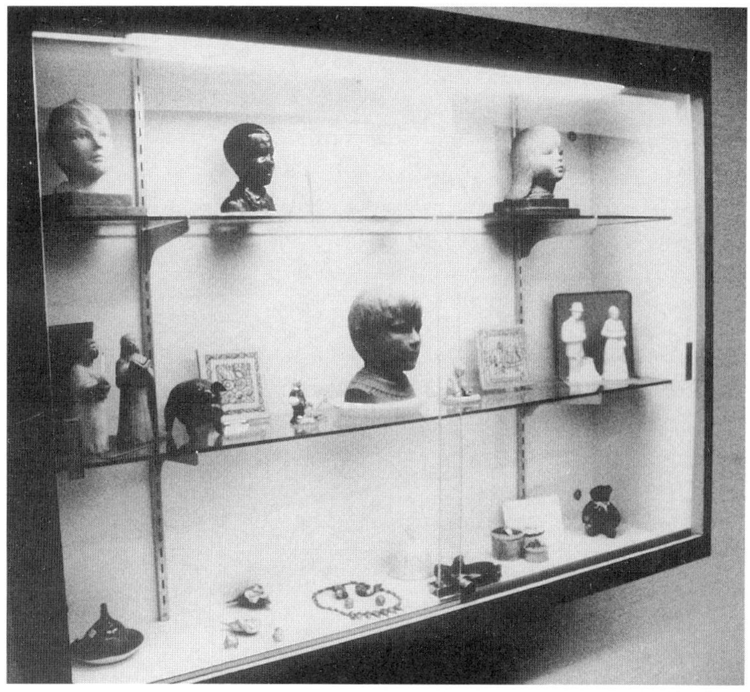

Display Case for Arts and Crafts (lower level of Central)

The greenhouse, which had been built on to the lower level, allows the horticulturists and flower arrangers to cultivate their skills, which in turn gives pleasure to everyone. A plant sale is held every spring and is also part of the arts and crafts fair in the fall.

Many of the details of daily living are organized through the committees in the *practical mechanics* group which covers such things as calendar clearance, guest and meeting room reservations, emergency food preparation and a fire brigade.

Another important service in this group is that of keeping the several bulletin boards up-to-date. There is space on one or the other of them for practically every facet of daily living in the community: bus schedules, current events, various classes, exercise programs, hospitalization of residents and announcements of every kind. There is a nature bulletin board which covers the happenings of nature on the campus, and a current events board.

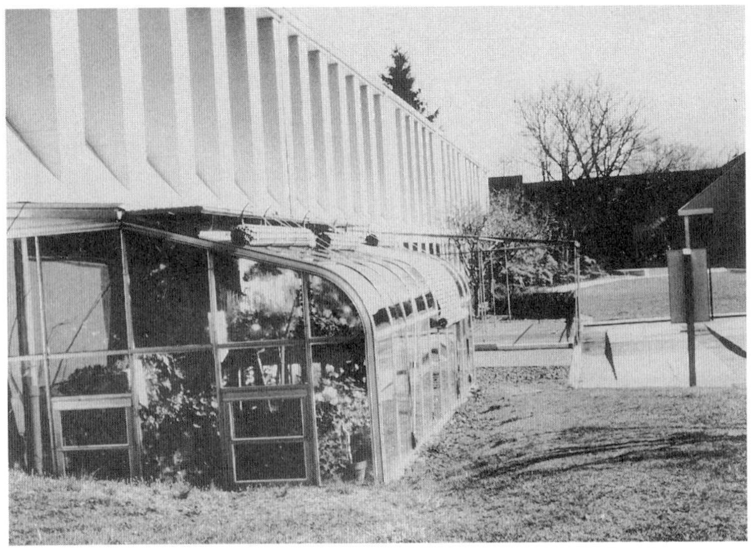

Greenhouse

Shuffleboard court to right. Dining room above.

It is through work on one or more of the *service* committees that an individual is able to go to bed at night with the satisfaction of knowing that he or she has helped someone else that day. It could be easy to feel worthless, living in a place where every need seems to be met, except for the fact that in an aging community there are always those who need an extra boost from time to time. Such things as the buddy system, helping the visually impaired, delivering Christmas packages and getting out the monthly *Bulletin* contribute to the well-being of all the residents.

The buddy system was organized and managed by a committee very soon after Foulkeways opened. Every person who lives alone in an apartment has a buddy. By eight A.M. the buddies are to have been in touch with each other. If a buddy doesn't answer the early morning call, the Health Center is alerted and someone goes to investigate. It is not a rarity that a serious consequence has been avoided because of the buddy system. When there are two persons sharing an apartment, either a husband and wife or two friends, they serve as each other's buddies.

The barn sales committee, which comes under services, serves a multiple purpose. The barn is a repository for everything that anyone at Foulkeways wants to dispose of. It is the first place to go if one is in need of something. It is the chief money-maker for the FRA. In 1990 the barn sales committee turned over $24,000 to the Residents' Association. Articles for the barn sales are outright gifts. The donor may get an appraisal for income tax purposes, but the money goes to the FRA.

All of the space on the upper level of the barn was eventually given over to the barn sales. Shelves were built, tables arranged and racks were installed for hanging things to make it possible to have attractive displays. While there are regular sale days during the summer, in the cold weather months it is necessary to have an appointment to visit the barn.

The largest group of all those who give service are the

Health Center volunteers. Approximately 120 workers are spread over twenty-one subcommittees. Some of the things they cover are: passing out juice and cookies in the afternoon, delivering mail to the rooms (and reading it when asked to do so), pushing wheelchairs to community events, running slide shows, conducting a weekly sing-along, and taking care of flowers and plants.

Three times a month a simple religious service is conducted in the upper lounge of Abington House. All of the Health Center residents who are able and want to come are helped to get there, where they all sit in a circle. The volunteer leader of the day uses selected readings, scriptural and otherwise, interspersed with four or five familiar hymns. The service lasts from twenty to thirty minutes and usually concludes with the Lord's Prayer.

Over four thousand hours per year of service are recorded by these volunteers. In manpower this amounts to two full-time employees. However, it is not possible to calculate the amount of satisfaction given and received through these efforts, nor the contribution that is made to the well-being of residents in the Health Center and in Abington House. Charles W. Lockyer, Jr. may have been thinking of all these things when he wrote in his letter of resignation from the board, (where he had been treasurer), "The employees and residents have been a delight to know. They testify to the goodness and greatness of which humanity is capable when persons care for and about each other."

This vast network of committees helps to make Foulkeways a pleasant, creative place to live. Moreover, the money the committees bring in is used to provide many extra things which add to the quality of life for everyone in the community. The electric beds in the Health Center were bought by the FRA, as were the individual television sets for each bed. The copier in the FRA office was paid for by the FRA. More than fifty thousand sheets of paper a year are copied free by residents. An electric typewriter was purchased for residents' use and in 1989 the washers and dryers, which had cost residents twenty-five cents per load to use, were made available at no cost to the user. After the swimming pool was built, the FRA purchased two automatic lifts to facilitate getting in and out of the pool for handicapped residents. Although there are alarm bells in every bathroom and an alarm goes off in Central when a telephone is off the hook, there is still the possibility that a resident might slip and fall while away from either of the two systems. In 1990 the FRA purchased a hundred pendant alarms which were given to any resident who felt the need of one. The pendant is operative within two hundred feet of a telephone.

A beautiful wall hanging which names all the committees of Foulkeways was designed and made by two residents, Frances McKee and Marguerite Spillman Wyttenbach. It hangs at the landing of the steps going from the upper to the lower level of Central.

The influence of the FRA extends beyond the confines of the Foulkeways campus. It encourages its members to write letters to government officials on issues having to do with the aging and other matters, and to go to township meetings when important matters concerning the larger community arise. The residents started a recycling program for newspapers, aluminum, glass and plastics before this became a township concern, and they are active in other environmental and conservation programs.

The importance of good physical health is regularly emphasized among the residents. Exercise classes — which include square dancing, ballet, and tap dancing — are led by experts from the resident body, and are held for every degree of physical competence and endurance. Outdoor games and competitions are organized and enthusiastically played. The two most popular exercises are walking on the well-kept paths and swimming in the exercise pool.

Part of the strength of Foulkeways' wonderful community spirit has its roots in the way new residents are received. As soon as new residents move in, a sponsor is

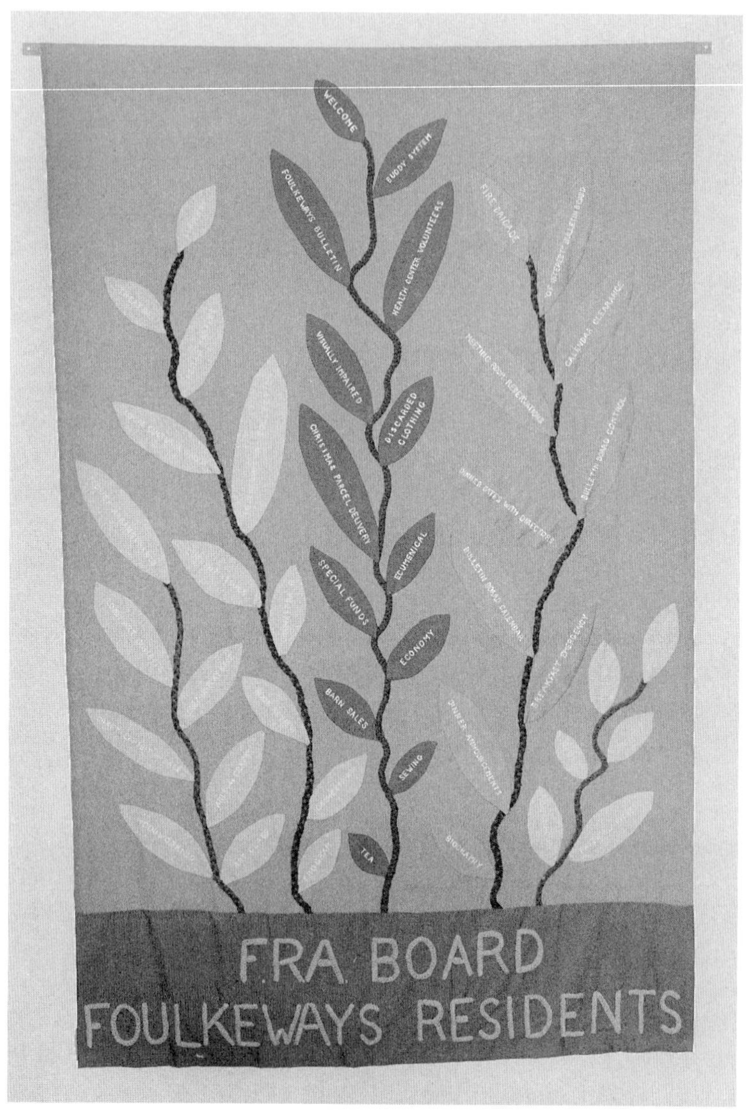

Wall Hanging

Each leaf represents a committee of the Foulkeways Residents' Association.

appointed to be responsible for making the transition as easy as possible for them. Plans are made for different people to have dinner with the new residents every night for the first week. As soon as they have settled in a bit, they are invited, but not urged, to find an agreeable activity in which to participate. In this way, they very quickly feel accepted as a contributing member in the life and work of the community. Equally important, the need that some residents might have to do nothing is respected, for no one is pushed against his or her wishes to do anything.

It can truthfully be said that all of the needs of an individual can be met at Foulkeways — the physical, intellectual, social, and spiritual. A meeting for worship, after the manner of Friends, is held every Sunday in the auditorium at Foulkeways. It had its origin on the first Sunday after opening day and continues with twenty-five to fifty in attendance. Some local churches arrange transportation for their members and car pools are planned by the residents themselves.

The Foulkeways administration is responsible for the physical needs of the residents. They take excellent care of the health of the residents and maintain the beauty and proper functioning of the grounds and the facilities. However, it is the residents, through the FRA and the various committees, who round out the days and fill up the hours with stimulating and enriching things to see and do. As one resident said as she scanned one of the bulletin boards, "They don't leave us much spare time, do they?"

THE ADMINISTRATION

Donald Moon quickly and efficiently settled into his work as the executive director of Foulkeways in 1978. He had made good use of the time he spent as Allen White's associate in becoming acquainted with the people, both residents and employees, and with the philosophy of Foulkeways. He formulated some ideas and plans during this time and was eager to rise to the challenge of running the retirement community.

One of his first ventures was to work with the board of directors on a revision of the life care agreement. Few changes were made, however. The original agreement had served as a model for other retirement communities in the area and needed little changing.

Within six months after taking office, Don was faced with reorganizing his office force when Richard Bansen resigned to become the associate secretary of general services of the Philadelphia Yearly Meeting. The search for an administrator to replace Dick Bansen provided seventy-five applicants, but none of these was hired. By shifting the responsibilities around, the running of Foulkeways was handled successfully without an administrator for the next few years. Karen Strawoet was employed in May 1979 as director of finance. She was also made officer in charge whenever the executive director had to be absent. Michael Peasley was moved from maintenance to become director of resident services. The installation of a computer in April 1979 added to the efficiency of the institution.

While he was reorganizing his staff, Donald Moon was also working on what he outlined as goals and directions of the future. Over several board meetings, he presented a comprehensive forty-page report on what he saw as important for every aspect of the life and administration of Foulkeways.

An early and major concern of Donald Moon's was the Residents' Assistance Fund. A fund had been started with specified bequests before Don took over but he, rightly, wanted it to grow. He set $500,000 as a goal to be reached by 1988 and a million dollars by 1998. Undoubtedly the goal served as a magnet for funds, for in just five years' time, by December 1983, the fund reached $515,607; by January 1992 it was over one and a half million dollars. The fund continues to grow through bequests in the wills of many residents and through various stipulated contributions. These funds are to assist persons already living at Foulkeways. However, administration has been apprised of future bequests of funds to be used specifically to help with entry fees for future applicants.

During Don's administration, a self-evaluation study was conducted by Nancy Gold and Karen Strawoet. They polled the residents and the corporate board members on what they liked about Foulkeways, what they would like to have changed, and what (if anything) they thought was special about it. There was an amazing similarity in the answers from the two groups, which pointed up how closely the board members related to the Foulkeways residents.

The residents repeatedly emphasized their awareness of a pervasive atmosphere of a simple, quiet elegance they felt in the life at Foulkeways. Together with the beautiful campus, this added up to a high degree of satisfaction. They also gave high marks for the comfort of the concept of continuing care, the independence enjoyed by the residents, and the special quality, (heard so frequently that it almost became hackneyed) referred to as the "spirit of Foulkeways." One resident stated that the questionnaire itself reflected the high standards the administration held, for, said she, "Foulkeways must constantly seek to avoid stagnation by questioning [its] mission as a home for several hundred persons."

It was at this time of self-study, however, that some questions among the residents came to the fore. Although residents who lived in the new apartments which were built on the seven-acre tract had been pleasantly assimilated into the community, some of the old-timers were uneasy about the future. If the board enlarged the community once, would they do it again? There were some who felt that the residents should have more input into the decisions relating to their daily lives. To quell this uneasiness and deal with future concerns, Richard Willis, president of the board, recommended in January 1981 that a Joint Advisory Council, similar to the one for the Health Center, be formed to make for better communication between the residents, the board, and administration. The council was to consist of one board member, who would be the chair, three representatives from administration, (namely, the executive director, the administrator, and the director of admissions), and three residents appointed by the president of the FRA. The minutes of the board of directors of November 1986 stated that the council "provides good contact and links of communication among the residents."

From the time back in January 1978, when residents were allowed to have dinner in the cafeteria, it was obvious that it was too small. In 1989, eleven years later, it was enlarged from a seating capacity of thirty-six to ninety-five. This could not have been done before the swimming pool complex was built, since it was necessary to move the laundry and housekeeping offices out of the main building to make room for the expansion of the Coffee Shop.

The plans were for lunch and dinner to be served to residents there on an optional basis. However breakfast, for those who took it, was to be served in the coffee shop instead of in the dining room. After several small meetings failed to satisfy objections to this decision, a larger meeting was held with members of the advisory council, some other invited persons, including several board members, and a delegation from the objecting residents. The matter was resolved by making all three meals available in both the coffee shop and the dining room. Following the breakfast dispute, the board of directors invited the president of the FRA to attend designated board meetings and, by request, any others he or she felt were necessary for good communication between the residents and the board.

The board had expressed its stand in relation to the FRA, and thereby to all residents, in September 1979 in the following terms:

> It is the intention of the Board of Directors that the Residents' Association should function as an independent and autonomous organization apart from the Corporate structure of Foulkeways at Gwynedd, the executive officers of the Corporation and the employees. Actions, including policy, will, however be subject to ratification by the Administration or the Board of Directors.

As early as 1982 Donald Moon began to look beyond the boundaries of Foulkeways. He and Richard Willis formed a committee called Friends Service for the Aging to explore possibilities for lower cost alternatives to the life-care concept. The committee would apply for grants to make feasibility studies in the field. Don worked up a mission statement which was recorded in the minutes of the board of directors in September 1984. It stated:

> [Our mission] is to explore the quality of life of older people in the most appropriate ways whether they are current residents, future residents or other elderly to whom we can provide services. This remains our mission today.

With the mission statement as a springboard, Donald Moon began to get more and more involved with activities in Friends Services for the Aging. Along with the board, he organized two separate corporations, one a consulting service called FRC Management, Inc., and the other to research life-care-at-home possibilities. Several members of the Foulkeways board were directors of one or the other of the new corporations. In September 1984 the Life-Care-at-Home Corporation joined forces with Jeanes Hospital and was called the Jeanes/Foulkeways Corporation. As the work of the new activities increased, more office space was required for them. In June 1986 Donald Moon moved to an office suite in nearby Springhouse, Pennsylvania. From there he continued to serve as the executive director of Foulkeways and as the president of the other two corporations.

There had been no administrator at Foulkeways since Richard Bansen left in 1979. That post was filled by assistants covering various areas. When Karen Strawoet, who had been Donald Moon's assistant, resigned in January 1983, Michael Peasley was moved into that position. Michael left in November 1985 to take a position at Meadowood, a new CCRC in the area. With Don's increasing outside responsibilities, it now became evident that Foulkeways needed a full time administrator. A search committee recruited, and the board was pleased to accept, Douglas A. Tweddale as the new administrator of Foulkeways. Douglas and his wife, Verna, arrived in January 1986 from Richmond, Indiana, where Doug had been the director of a hospice home care program. In keeping with Foulkeways tradition, they were welcomed at a reception given by the residents shortly after their arrival.

Doug served as administrator of Foulkeways until July 1990 when he became the executive director. Don, who had been executive director for twelve years, had given notice that he would like to resign so he could have more time for his other interests, especially the Jeanes/Foulkeways Corporation and FRC Management, Inc. These two corporations were legally separated from Foulkeways shortly afterward, and they were renamed Friends Life Care at Home, and Friends Retirement Concepts respectively. The board, even as it regretted to see Don go, enthusiastically endorsed Doug as Don's successor.

The staff and residents showed their affection and

appreciation for Donald and Carolyn Moon at a large farewell party which was held in the auditorium of Central. The board expressed its gratitude for Don's leadership in a resolution where he was thanked for "... faithfully preserving and enhancing the spirit of Foulkeways that makes our community second to none."

Douglas Tweddale was well-qualified to hold the reins as executive director of Foulkeways, due to his four-year stint as administrator. He had been certified as a nursing home administrator by the Commonwealth of Pennsylvania in June 1987. Since Doug had a strong office staff, the need for another administrator was not pressing, so that post, again, was not filled.

The office staff increased considerably between the early days and 1990. At that time Sue McMullen and Sandra Smith, secretaries, and Charles B. Ermentrout, comptroller, made up the office force along with Allen White, executive director, and Robert Trier, administrator. When Doug Tweddale became executive director in July 1990, the office force had expanded to include, along with the above, a maintenance secretary, a medical/health insurance coordinator, a payroll/personnel secretary, and a personnel director.

The reception area, which is the first thing to be seen inside the front door, is the pivot of Central. The receptionists see all and know everything that happens at Foulkeways — or so the residents appear to believe. The receptionists not only operate the telephone exchange from seven in the morning until nine in the evening, they get out of their chairs a million (more or less) times a day to get things out of, or put something into, the residents' individual message boxes. And they do it all with a smile.

Early in January 1991, a five-year consulting committee was appointed to study strategies for the future of Foulkeways. There were twelve members on the committee, coming from staff, residents and the board. The committee was instructed to study trends in other CCRCs and to determine how Foulkeways might be improved to assure its future viability.

Studies showed that the demand for studio apartments was diminishing, that prospective residents wanted more space in the one-bedroom apartments and that the demand for two-bedroom apartments was increasing. After months of research, the committee recommended that twelve new two-bedroom apartments be built and that twelve more be created by combining twelve studio with twelve one-bedroom apartments. This "add twelve, take twelve" was to satisfy an earlier commitment (made in 1980) that no more new apartments would be built at Foulkeways. The committee also recommended that some of the one-bedroom apartments be enlarged by incorporating the patio into the living room which would create more living and storage space in those apartments. The committee was convinced that these changes were necessary to keep Foulkeways in a competitive position in the market.

All of those involved realized they were dealing with a sensitive area. Nothing is so unsettling as change, and many residents said they did not want Foulkeways to get any bigger. The mission statement had been revised in 1990 to read as follows:

> The mission of Foulkeways at Gwynedd is to provide community life for elderly persons desiring to maintain or improve their quality of life and security within a framework of mutual caring and Quaker ideals.

With this statement, plus the earlier commitment to build no more apartments, the board was under the weight of finding a way to keep residents satisfied, while at the same time, securing the financial stability of Foulkeways. Two Quaker issues were involved: that of living up to their responsibility and that of achieving unity among the constituents before an action is taken.

Some residents thought there might be more demand for the studio apartments if the entry fee could be reduced or, if not that, then perhaps the entry fee could be subsidized for worthy individuals who needed it. Either of these might make it possible for teachers, social workers, librarians, nurses, or others who have led lives of service to have the comfort and security of Foulkeways, and this would help to keep the studio apartments occupied.

Others were against the building of any new apartments. Some living in the one-bedroom apartments were in favor of having them enlarged; others who lived in them did not want to be disturbed. Letters of protest were written to the five-year consulting committee and a well-attended meeting of the residents to discuss the situation was held in the auditorium in September, 1991. The decision reached at that time was to hold off on any new construction and to delay any doubling up of apartments. A prototype of the enlarged one-bedroom apartment would be constructed for residents to inspect.

The matter has not yet been permanently resolved. However, the priority list remains a barometer of the health of the institution and everyone agrees that anything which affects that health must be evaluated carefully.

Meanwhile, plans to celebrate the twenty-fifth anniversary of the opening of Foulkeways were well under way. The celebrations every five years had been joyous occasions, but the silver anniversary observance on November 10, 1992 must be a very special one. Committees were appointed in the summer of 1991 to plan every detail. The residents who had come in during the first six months of Foulkeways existence would be honored at the celebration, as would those who had worked so hard to get it built.

CENTRAL

The office wing of Central had been re-arranged, painted and re-carpeted in 1977. Preliminary studies had been done at that time for upgrading all of Central with special emphasis on enlarging the auditorium but other matters were more pressing. In September 1980 a facility expansion committee was appointed to study future needs of Foulkeways and make recommendations. This committee reaffirmed the principles which the board had previously established. They were:

a. That Foulkeways build no more apartments nor any other projects which would substantially increase the total number of residents who live under our life care agreement.
b. That any future building plans should be considered only insofar as they increase the Central facilities to our residents.
c. That any future building be done only after the need has been clearly established.
d. That any physical additions or improvements to Foulkeways which are non-income producing be financed through contributions.

With these principles in mind, the expansion committee then recommended the following:

> [to build] an elevator, an expanded auditorium, an arts/activities area, a central library, and a swimming pool.
>
> The committee also recommends that the administration continue with plans to upgrade the one-bedroom apartments through the expansion of the

> kitchen units and the addition of a storage area. The financing of these additions (to the apartments) will be covered by additional entry fees to these apartments.

Architects from the firm of Ewing, Cole, Erdman & Eubank were engaged to submit plans for all these changes and additions, excluding the pool, and the fundraisers went into action. Donald Moon was able to report to the board in January 1982 that $986,086 had been raised from cash pledges and outstanding bequests. The estimated costs for the proposed improvements was $900,000. The building contract was signed with the George H. Baver Company and ground breaking was set for March.

The auditorium was enlarged by forty feet, with a dressing room on each side of the now-adequate stage, as well as more seating space for the audiences. It was ready in time for the fifteenth anniversary celebration of Foulkeways that November, and was inaugurated with a piano recital on a new Baldwin grand piano.

The new library was put on the lower level of Central. A games room, with space for a pool table and card tables, was also on the lower level. There was room for a large carpeted multi-purpose room to be used for special parties, as an exercise room and as an indoor Wimbledon court. A hard-surfaced area was created for a shuffleboard court. Space for a branch bank, which would be open three days a week, was also found on the lower level. The newly installed elevator made both levels accessible to all of the residents, regardless of handicaps.

By the beginning of 1991, all of Central had been remodeled and redecorated. New wall coverings and carpets were installed in the main lobby. The adjacent dining room also had new wall and floor treatments and all of the chairs had been refinished and re-upholstered. The front entrance to Central, redesigned to include a *porte cochere*, was done over at the same time as the redecorating of Central and the walkways adjacent to Central were resurfaced with an attractive finish. Foulkeways, well into its third decade, looked fresh and new, belying its twenty-four years of constant activity.

THE HEALTH CENTER

The Health Center was running smoothly when Donald Moon became executive director in 1978. He was registered as a nursing home administrator in the Commonwealth of Pennsylvania in January 1979. In April 1981 the Health Center committee of the board of directors was asked to consider improvements to the Health Center. It recommended that the out-patient clinic area be expanded to include an additional examining room, an office for the resident care nurse, a staff development room which also served as an office for the assistant director of nurses. A room each for the director of nursing services and for the social service worker, along with a more adequate physical therapy room and a suitable waiting room for the out-patient clinic were included in the plans. Also under consideration was the creation of four or five more private rooms in Gwynedd House.

The architects who were designing the improvements to Central were asked to make drawings for the desired changes in the Health Center and the same builders were engaged. Donald Moon's successful fund raising efforts for Central covered the costs for the Health Center renovations. Ground was broken on March 1, 1982; an open house was held the following October. There was general satisfaction with the enlarged facility throughout the Health Center and this permeated the entire community. Residents were especially grateful for the addition of four private rooms in Gwynedd House.

In April 1980 James C. Alden, M.D. was appointed the medical director and primary physician for the Health Center and the whole community. He had no assistants at that time. In 1987 the medical set-up was reorganized. Dr.

Alden had asked to have his patient load reduced by half, so Lawrence Beck, M.D., was made the new medical director. The medical director has no patients but is responsible for and has oversight of all the medical care given at Foulkeways.

After the reorganization Dr. Alden was responsible for primary care for the Health Center and for out-patient care two days a week. Eileen Bonner, M.D. was in charge of Abington House and the entrance examinations. Margaret Simcox, M.D. took care of out-patients except for the two days per week when Dr. Alden was available.

There were many changes in the personnel of the Health Center in 1988. Dr. Beck resigned, after only a year, to take a position with the Geisinger Medical Center in Danville, Pennsylvania. He was replaced by Barbara Bell, M.D. The beloved Betty Cash, R.N. who had been the out-patient clinic nurse for twenty years retired. Lois Whittemore, R.N. was welcomed to replace her and continues, successfully, in that position. Gerri Paier, R.N., M.S.N., C.R.N.P., who had been engaged to assist Jane Kummerer Butler as nurse practitioner for Abington House and to do research for the Frank Morgan Jones Fund, left in August 1988 to enter a Ph.D. program in gerontological nursing at the University of Pennsylvania. The Frank Morgan Jones Fund of $250,000 had been set up by a resident, William H. Russell, in memory of his father-in-law, to finance studies in gerontology at Foulkeways in conjunction with the University of Pennsylvania's School of Nursing.

Jane Butler expressed a desire to resign her position as director of nursing services and to work only three days a week as a replacement for Gerri Paier in Abington House and with out-patients. Joyce Wallace, R.N., M.S.N., C.R.N.P. came on the Health Center staff in May 1990 to be available when Jane Butler was not on duty. Linda Boston, R.N., M.A., M.B.A. replaced Jane as the new director of nursing services in October 1988. She and Dr. Bell were welcomed at a tea in November. Linda established an excellent rapport with the residents of Foulkeways by visiting each person in his or her apartment during the early months of her tenure at Foulkeways.

As the Health Center expanded through the years, so did the services it provided. After training in psychotherapy, which enhanced her already good skills, Pat Miller became entitled to professionally sign her name as Patricia Miller, M.S.S., A.C.S.W., L.S.W. (Academy of Certified Social Workers. Licensed by Commonwealth of Pennsylvania.) The full-time pharmacist, currently Denise Lannon, R.P.H., works in enlarged quarters with a greater inventory than previously.

When Foulkeways was opened a physical therapist was on call, but there was very little equipment for this purpose at that time. Space for physical therapy had been allotted when the other wings were added in 1974, but a well-equipped physical therapy room was not available until the Health Center office wing was remodeled in 1982. Thomas B. Swartley, P.T., who had come to the staff as a full-time therapist in 1980, rejoiced in the new accommodations where he could more effectively treat the constant flow of patients who came from the resident body as well as from the Health Center.

At the unforgettable germinal meeting at Gwynedd Meeting on April 28, 1963, when William Clarke had breathed new life into the moribund Beaumont committee, Eleanor Clarke had stood up and said, "And there must be a swimming pool." Just twenty-five years later on August 4, 1988, an open house was held to celebrate the opening of the new exercise pool in a separate building called the Natatorium. After polling the residents to measure their interest in a pool, the administration, along with the board, decided that if the residents could raise $300,000 to be escrowed as an endowment to cover operating costs, the pool could be built with accumulated unrestricted bequest funds. Lynn Taylor Associates designed the pool complex which would house a new laundry, housekeeping offices, locker rooms with showers, and an exercise room as well as the 25×60×4½ foot exercise pool and a smaller, warmer therapy pool. C. Raymond Davis & Sons were awarded the contract to do the building.

A qualified pool director was hired and the pool quickly became a popular place. It was used not only for exercise but for games such as volleyball and for water ballet. The therapy pool was excellent for residents who needed hydrotherapy. The physical therapist could get into the pool with them and direct and assist in beneficial exercises.

An occupational therapist, Janet Bigley, is on call at the Health Center. Sue Schulz, a recreational therapist, is at Foulkeways as a full-time employee, along with her puppy, Snickers, who is considered the Health Center dog.

Snickers' coming to the Health Center is in accordance with the new thinking about pets. When Foulkeways opened, residents were allowed to bring pets if they already had them, but were not permitted to replace them. When gerontological studies began to show the therapeutic value of pets for older people, this ruling was changed. Now residents may acquire a pet at any time.

Beth Lynch, a recreational therapist who was engaged in an innovative new approach as a special services person, is also on a full-time basis. Beth, a recent college graduate, has a very flexible job description. The only solid directive for her is to spread cheer and feelings of happiness and well-being among the Health Center residents whenever and wherever she can. Regina Peasley, who later became a resident, was first employed in 1989 to visit residents who were hospitalized in neighboring hospitals who had no "significant other" living in the area.

The Health Center staff began a campaign in 1989 to do away with restraints for roving or restless patients. Within a year they could announce that Foulkeways was restraint-free. Research on this issue shows that physical restraints on a confused person only adds to his or her confusion. Through creative nursing techniques and thoughtful architectural planning, restraints can be avoided, thus adding to the well-being of the patient.

To keep patients from wandering outside, electronic sensors were put on the outside doors. Patients were furnished with plastic bracelets which ring a bell to alert the nurses when a patient wearing a bracelet goes through the door. To give these patients a greater sense of freedom and still have them protected, there are two enclosed gardens off the Health Center lounges. There are benches and tables in the gardens and also a little pond with a waterfall in one of them.

A charming episode about a confused patient who had wandered outside is told about Ron Foltz, head of the maintenance department. The nurse was having no success in persuading the patient to go inside. "Young lady," said the patient, "I'm over eighty years old. I don't need to be told by *you* what to do." Ron was passing by and sized up the situation. Looking up into the patient's face, he said, "A beautiful young woman like you needs a handsome escort." He offered his arm. She took it and together they walked into the Health Center.

This account of how the Health Center functions would not be complete if the two important support personnel who help keep things on an even keel were not mentioned. Currently, Leslie C. Jordan, the receptionist, is secretary to the director of nursing services (Linda Boston), and manages the switchboard of the Health Center. Lisa D. Cianci, ward clerk, holds things together in Gwynedd House, relieving the busy nurses of countless details.

As Foulkeways evolved into more and better quarters and services, the state licensing requirements also became more stringent. When the first residents moved in on that cold day in 1967, the only legal requirements for opening were for the executive director to be certified as an administrator of nursing homes by the Commonwealth of Pennsylvania, and that the Health Center pass state approval and certification by Medicare. As continuing care retirement communities (CCRCs) with the obligatory nursing care proliferated, more and more official scrutiny began to be turned on them.

Twenty years after its inception, the Health Center not only had to be certified annually by the Pennsylvania Department of Health through its Division of Long-Term Care, its Division of Safety, and its Department of Welfare, but the authority to function had to be granted again under the Continuing Care Provider Registration and Disclosure Act of 1984. This meant inspection by the Pennsylvania Insurance Department. Today the Bureau of Labor sees to it that fair hiring standards are met, as well as that safety precautions are enforced. The Health Center is regularly visited and inspected by Medicare teams and by the Pennsylvania Department of Welfare.

Over and above the legal requirements, Foulkeways now engages in a self-evaluation process every five years on a voluntary basis. In 1961, as a self-regulating mechanism for the mushrooming industry of care for the aging, the American Association of Homes for the Aging (AAHA) was organized in Washington, D.C. In 1985 a national accreditation program called the Continuing Care Accreditation Commission (CCAC) was developed under the aegis of AAHA.

This program calls for a comprehensive self-study exercise covering every major activity of a facility's operation. After the self-evaluation has been done, a committee from CCAC spends three days with those involved and the retirement center is appraised according to the carefully defined mission of the CCAC. The benefit of this process is two-fold: it helps the retirement center to discover its strengths and weaknesses, and the approval of the CCAC gives national recognition to the approved facility.

THE BOARD OF DIRECTORS

Richard B. Willis, president of the board of directors since 1975, successfully steered Foulkeways through the many changes in administration and in the physical organization of Foulkeways during his tenure of eleven years. Alterations were made in the one-bedroom units shortly after he took office. The kitchens were enlarged so that full-sized refrigerators could be put in and more closet space was created.

The priority list was an early concern for him as he watched Kendal, Crosslands and Cathedral Village draw off some of those on the Foulkeways waiting list. The proliferation of CCRCs in the area creates a challenge that is constantly monitored by the board of directors. However, Foulkeways is fortunate in that it has been able to maintain a satisfactory priority list in spite of the competition.

When Gwynedd Meeting gave the Beaumont committee permission to incorporate back in 1963, it stipulated that all of the members of the corporation be Quakers and the majority of them be members of Gwynedd Meeting. As it became evident that all of the special talents required for the competent handling of the affairs of Foulkeways could not be found within Quakerdom, the Foulkeways bylaws were amended in 1980 as follows:

> Article IX ... No less than 75 percent of the Board of Directors shall at all times be members of the Religious Society of Friends.

Even though the majority of the directors were no longer members of Gwynedd Meeting, the Meeting was happy about its relationship with Foulkeways. This was borne out by its reaction to the concern which Albert Maris raised in December 1980 regarding the 99-year lease which Foulkeways had with Gwynedd Meeting. He saw that there could be a problem when the termination date of 2065 A.D. approached.

The lease, signed in 1966, had been devised in order to give Gwynedd Meeting a means of recovering the property in case the "new and untried venture" should fail. Said Albert Maris, as reported in Gwynedd Meeting's monthly minutes:

> Thirteen years of successful and financially sound operation should now dispel that fear, however, while the prospect of having to surrender the leased land in 2060 will present for many years before that date a major obstacle to accepting new residents for lifetime care.

Albert Maris, William Pye, and Samuel Swansen, with Richard Willis as an ex-officio member, were appointed to approach Gwynedd Meeting about the matter. They were instructed to ask the Meeting to transfer to Foulkeways the title of the leased 70.353 acres on which Foulkeways was built, either outright as a gift or for money, and also to convey the title of the 3.4 acres southwest of Abington House to Foulkeways. This parcel had been bought and paid for by Foulkeways in 1964 before Foulkeways became incorporated. The original sixty-four acres of farmland had been increased to sixty-seven by the addition of the three acres on Sumneytown Pike which the Meeting had bought in 1951. The ground around the Lowry house was added when Foulkeways was built, bringing the total acreage in the leasehold to over seventy acres.

At Gwynedd's monthly meeting in February 1981, Gwynedd Meeting appointed Rolland H. Henderson, Mary Edna Zimmerman Ott, Robert M. Russell II and C. Edward Zimmerman as a committee to study the request, with Richard Willis an ex-officio member.

There was no problem about the title to the 3.4 acres.

It was transferred without question. The case of the ground lease was another matter. The two committees — the one from Foulkeways and the one from Gwynedd Meeting — wrestled with the problem for a period of two years. There were some in the Meeting who felt that by giving away the land they would be subsidizing persons who could well afford to pay; others countered with, "But there are many who cannot afford it, and we are concerned about them." There were those who thought that by selling it, the Meeting's memorial to May Foulke Beaumont would be sullied.

Underneath all the explorations was the recurring sense of Gwynedd Meeting's feeling of being blessed by its connection to Foulkeways and the desire to retain the relationship. After two years of searching, unity in the Meeting was reached. In January 1983 Gwynedd Meeting agreed that it would amend the existing lease by adding a provision for the automatic extension of the lease for additional terms of 99 years, if at the end of the previous term Foulkeways was continuing to use the leased property exclusively for the housing and care of the elderly. The Gwynedd monthly meeting Minutes of January 1983 record the following:

> Strong feelings of support for Foulkeways were expressed as well as the desire that its continued operation as long as possible and desirable be assured by the Meeting as proposed by the committee. At the same time, satisfaction was expressed that under the committee's proposal the present close relationship between the Meeting and Foulkeways would remain unchanged. Foulkeways' Board of Directors, staff and residents include a great many members of the Meeting. The hope was expressed that these close ties would be continued and increased.

Foulkeways' board of directors was satisfied with the outcome and expressed its appreciation to Albert Maris for his foresight and to Gwynedd Meeting for its interest and generosity.

Foulkeways already had protected itself along its eastern boundary by buying the seven-acre tract, but it was in a vulnerable position along the north-western property line. There was a possibility that in the future the corner where Route 202 crosses Sumneytown Pike would be zoned for commercial use. To circumvent such a threat to Foulkeways, the board decided to buy the properties in that area as they came on the market. The first house to be acquired was that of Graham and Grace Smith (who later became residents) on Sumneytown Pike in 1987. The Toth house next door to the Smith house was purchased in 1989 and the O'Hara property, on Meetinghouse Road adjacent to the post office, was also bought in 1989. This gave Foulkeways control of the corner with the exception of only one remaining house. Foulkeways was able to get an option to buy that one whenever it comes on the market in the future.

The Smith house was made into a two-bedroom apartment on the first floor and two much-needed guest suites were created on the second floor. The Toth house was left as a single-family residence, as was the O'Hara house. The acquisition of these properties, together with the leased ground, brought the total of Foulkeways real estate holdings to 94 acres.

The new houses were named in accordance with the custom of naming the other sections of Foulkeways for important Friends who were no longer living. By ballot, they were named White (for Allen White, Foulkeways' first executive director), Woolman, and Walton.

Alan Hunt, who had served Foulkeways so faithfully from its beginning as legal counsel, felt obliged to resign in April 1986 because he was on the board and was counsel for Kendal. The board expressed its gratitude to Alan for his fine service and welcomed William A. Humenuk, Esq. as a replacement.

In May 1986, Richard Willis presented his resignation as president of the board. He had been an officer of the Foulkeways board since 1965 when he succeeded Thomas

Elkinton as treasurer. The board designated him President Emeritus and expressed its appreciation to him for his twenty-one years of service as follows:

> During his tenure as President many advances have been made by the Corporation which uniquely bear the imprint of his influence. The Board expressed its gratitude ... for the influence of his character which will live on beyond his years of tenure as President of the Corporation.

Samuel T. Swansen, Esq., who had come on the board in March 1979, was appointed the new president.

GENERAL SERVICES

There are four components in a continuing care retirement community. They are the corporate board, the administration, the resident body, and general services. Foulkeways is not only a well-kept campus with interesting residents and wonderful health care, it is also a place which requires a great deal of tending. The services which make all of the good things possible are the connective tissue which holds the structure together.

Ronald S. Foltz came to Foulkeways as director of maintenance in 1985 to replace Herbert Myers, who had taken over when Michael Peasley became one of Don Moon's assistants. Ron is ultimately responsible for the whole physical establishment, inside and out. He puts in a long day and is on call twenty-four hours a day. He is in charge of security, transportation, upkeep, and any and all of the day-by-day emergencies which arise. He and his staff are at the beck and call of the residents to do such things as replace a light bulb, or to help take a load of things to or from a storage area. They also man the electric carts which transport residents who need assistance to and from apartments to Central or the Health Center. All requests from residents to maintenance must go through Margaret Wood, the maintenance secretary.

The pleasant campus — with its great variety of evergreen and deciduous trees, its flowering shrubs, its spacious lawns, and lovely flower beds — is the special responsibility of Thomas C. Daley, who has a B.S. in ornamental horticulture. The walking paths through the woods which surround the campus on three sides are under his watchful eye. Tom and his assistants keep the tiny stream which flows alongside the Abington House woods and under the Japanese bridge free of debris. The grass Wimbledon courts are kept in top-notch condition. The active grounds committee of the FRA aids and abets Tom and his staff in their endeavors to make Foulkeways ever more appealing. All this and more: Tom is gifted with a chain saw. Scattered through the wooded areas are weathered wooden owls, rabbits, ducks

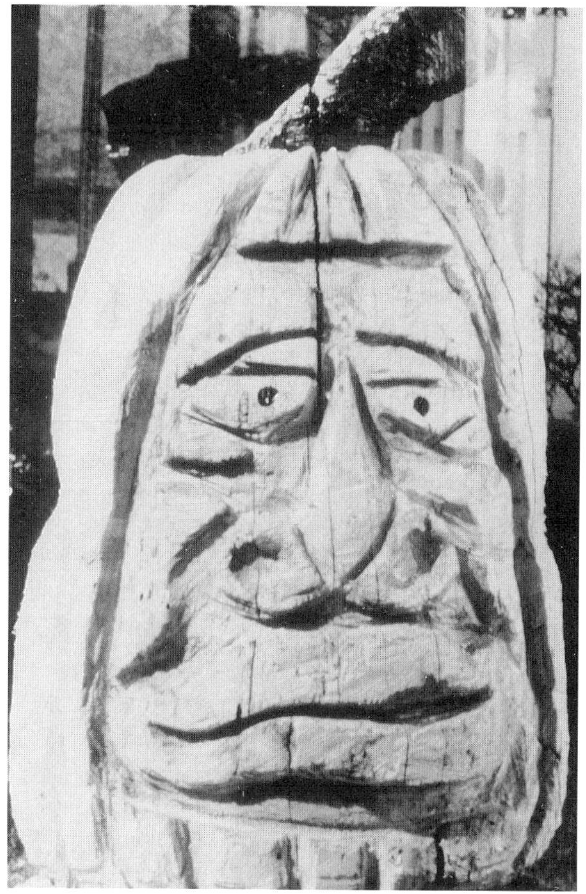

Jack-O'-Lantern

One of several sculptures created by Tom Daley with a chain saw.

and Pooh Bear, who guards the Bear Crossing at the Maris Trail in the south woods. He even made large wooden jack-o'-lanterns which he puts out at Halloween. All of these Tom has created solely with a chain saw from logs and stumps.

Unremitting and herculean efforts are required to keep Foulkeways clean, shining and welcoming. Cynthia Prediger, currently director of housekeeping, is responsible for all housekeeping details. All public areas are cleaned daily and all apartments are done weekly. Since all linens are furnished, not only in the Health Center but for all apartments, it is the responsibility of the housekeeping department to see that they are in plentiful supply and good condition.

Food Service is second only to the Health Center in importance as far as the residents are concerned. The current director of food service is Roberta Isbell, B.S., R.D. She works under the Culinary Service Network, an outside service which was founded by Chip Kent and Gene Dollof, both of whom had worked at Foulkeways as food service managers under Stouffer's. Robbie has a closing manager, a food production manager, and a dietitian as assistants. Approximately seven hundred meals are served daily by the food staff. The greatest proportion of these are dinners for, except for those in the Health Center, few residents take more than one meal a day in the main dining room.

There are two dining room managers, one for Abington House and one for the main dining room, and, presently, two hostesses. For over twenty years Anna Pearl Hostetler was the hostess in the main dining room. The atmosphere of dignified dining was developed under her supervision, for she had the responsibility of training the young servers as they came and went. This she did with a firm but loving hand. There are over a hundred part-time servers employed, most of whom come from local high schools and colleges. There appears to be a mutual admiration society between the residents and these fresh-faced young people.

LOOKING AHEAD

Continuing care retirement communities have come a long way since Foulkeways first opened its doors in 1967, almost twenty-five years ago. It was the first such community in Pennsylvania and the second in the Delaware Valley. (Meadow Lakes, in Hightstown, New Jersey, opened a short time before Foulkeways.) It was soon followed by two other Quaker life-care communities, Kendal in Kennett Square, Pennsylvania, and Medford Leas in Medford, New Jersey. At the end of 1991, there were forty-six CCRCs within a radius of fifty miles of Philadelphia, the largest concentration in the United States and in the world. Seven are Quaker sponsored. Many are church sponsored, nonprofit institutions, although more are being built and run for profit by big businesses such as the Marriott Corporation, which operates the Quadrangle in Haverford, Pennsylvania.

The management of CCRCs is a new and growing industry. In a report to the board of directors in September 1986, Donald Moon pointed out that creating and administering retirement communities has become big business. Colleges are offering courses in CCRC management.

With the increasing percentage of older citizens in the population, it appears that the momentum already generated toward retirement centers will continue to foster this growth industry for some time into the future. There will be keen competition among the various centers to attract new residents and to keep their priority lists in a healthy condition.

Everyone connected with Foulkeways believes that what Foulkeways has to offer will continue to have strong appeal to the aging population. Foulkeways is fortunate to have at this time a young, strong, and able executive director who is consistent and caring. Douglas Tweddale has proven his ability to meet the challenge of trying to keep the diverse group of residents happy and satisfied, while at the same time doing what must be done for the good of the community. One of his strong points is in keeping the lines of communication open; in true Quaker tradition he allows each individual to be heard. His cheerful countenance and ready smile give residents a feeling of confidence and contribute much to the pleasant atmosphere of Foulkeways.

The hope is that the spacious, well-kept campus, the regulated size of the resident body, and the special quality of friendly interaction among the several components of Foulkeways will continue to attract new residents and keep Foulkeways as it has been for a quarter of a century: a vibrant, happy place to live out one's years, creatively and productively.

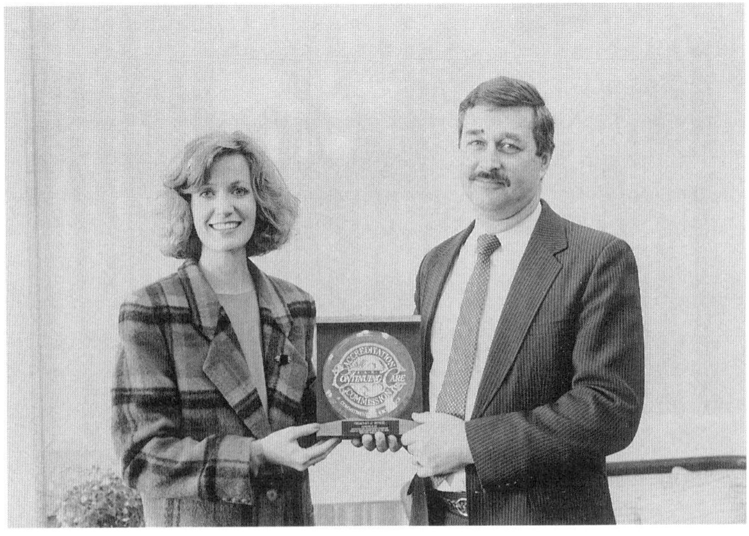

Anne Gillespie, from the Continuing Care Accreditation Committee, presenting plaque to Executive Director Douglas Tweddale, February 12, 1992.

IN CONCLUSION

Foulkeways at Gwynedd carries out a dream of Gwynedd Friends Meeting ... to [create] a community planned for older citizens where ... people could find persons of common interest and comparable age with whom to share the mature friendship and mutual support that only the rich experiences of a lifetime make possible.

— *Harry Sprogell (1912–1972)*

The Treasure and the Dream. As a resident commented, what a satisfaction it must have been to the founders to see that the treasure was indeed well-used when the dream became a reality.

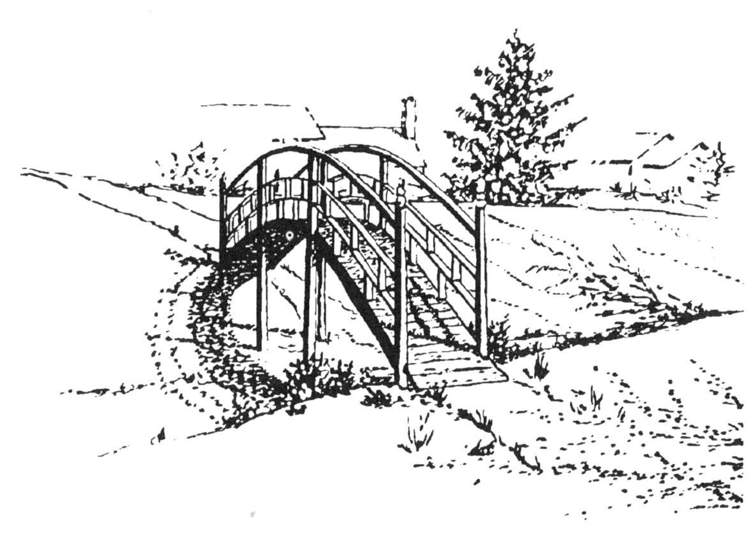

Appendices

APPENDIX A

HOW TO CHOOSE THE CONTINUING CARE COMMUNITY THAT IS RIGHT FOR YOU

As you approach retirement age are you anxious about what your later years will bring? Where you will be? Who will take care of you if or when you need it? How adequate your plans for financial security might be? What would happen should you need to be in a nursing home for several months, or even years?

Continuing care retirement communities (CCRCs) are the contemporary places to live in peace, security, and contentment as one grows old in a turbulent world. They can help to solve the current problem of caring for, and being cared for, in a society that no longer produces cohesive families. They can provide security from the costs of catastrophic illness and furnish some measure of financial and personal safety. They can offer the newest and best way of independent living for those who would avoid nursing homes or moving in with an overburdened relative.

Within the last twenty-five years, retirement communities have become a large and growing industry. Before 1970 there were only two continuing care communities on the east coast — one in New Jersey and one in Pennsylvania. From coast to coast throughout the United States and Canada, more than seven hundred nonprofit CCRCs now exist, with many more under construction. Many CCRCs are under the care of various religious groups; some are being built and managed by big corporations. As is to be expected, quality and stability vary greatly from one facility to another.

As a consumer, you should investigate your choices carefully before making your selection. Reading and analyzing literature and visiting selected sites is time-consuming, but necessary. You can't count on getting in such a facility when you have a crisis, *so you must plan ahead.*

Since the better places have waiting (or priority) lists, application to a chosen facility should be made well ahead of the time of desired occupancy — two or three years at the very least. This means that your initial investigation of CCRCs should begin quite a bit earlier.

A *National Continuing Care Directory* put out by the American Association of Homes for the Aging (AAHA) is available in bookstores and libraries. You can select possible CCRCs from it, then write for brochures for more detailed study. You can obtain more information by calling AAHA in Washington D.C. at (202) 783-2242.

Here are the eight most important things to consider when looking at Continuing Care Communities:

1. Location
2. Attitude of Residents
3. Living Accommodations
4. Health Care
5. Services
6. Resident Activities
7. Management Philosophy
8. Financial Status

Location

The geographical location of an acceptable community is very important. Climate is a big consideration for many. Some want to enjoy the changing of the seasons; others prefer a warmer area.

Proximity to children is desirable, but this should not be the sole deciding factor in choosing a retirement community. Young people are susceptible to being here today and somewhere else tomorrow.

If a well-qualified CCRC exists in one's own community, the bonus of old ties and friendships, familiarity with roads, shopping areas, and other services should not be discounted.

The surrounding or larger community should be looked

at. Is the retirement community near what is important to you? For many, this means a city where there are concert halls, museums, theaters and sports. How are the medical facilities in that area? Is there a college nearby? Does the local community show signs of a well-run progressive government?

Attitude of Residents

The best way to make a judgment about the attitude of the residents is to visit the CCRCs you selected. It is best to make an appointment, but there is nothing wrong with just dropping in. The general atmosphere of a facility reflects the attitude of those who live there as well as those who administer the place. Talk to residents. Ask them what they like about their lives there. Observe interactions between residents, between residents and employees, and between residents and administration. Does this appear to be a friendly, cooperative community or is it more like an exclusive resort? Is it compatible with your own lifestyle?

Living Accommodations

To move from a house full of treasured belongings into an apartment of any size is a traumatic experience, both emotionally and physically. However, it can also be the beginning of a life free of the burden of too many things to look after. In a retirement community where there are plenty of opportunities for creative living, the size of the apartment is not so important as long as it is adequate for your needs.

More important than the size of the apartments are the standards of upkeep of the general facility. Cleanliness and order, indoors and out, are exceedingly important for happy, contented living. A well-planned and well-operated facility will have these qualities in good measure. The apartments should look out onto pleasant surroundings; the public rooms should be tastefully furnished, arranged, and well-cared for. The campus should be beautiful and inviting.

If a facility appeals to you, try to spend some time there. If staying a few days is out of the question, at least have a meal there. The atmosphere of the dining room and the quality of the meals are important. You will probably be living in the CCRC for the rest of your life.

Health Care

Most people go to a continuing care community for the guaranteed health care; therefore, the health center is of prime concern. Visit it. Observe the residents living there. Are they out of bed, dressed and unrestrained? Is the place clean? Is there a feeling of order? Is it free of offensive odors? Is it a place where you would like to receive care?

What are the levels of care? Is there a personal care unit for those who need supervision but do not yet need skilled care? What about those with Alzheimer's or other mental illnesses? Is there a place for them? Do the nurses and attendants seem to be kind and considerate? Is a doctor always available? Again, ask questions of the residents in the health center while you are looking around.

Other Services

What services, other than health care, are offered? Is the apartment cleaned on a weekly basis and are linens furnished? Is extra help available if a resident needs or desires it? Is there transportation for shopping and other services for those who can no longer drive? Are there guest rooms available for visitors?

Resident Activities

Is there an activities director or do the residents plan their own programs? The communities where the residents do their own planning appear to have a greater sense of fellowship than those where it is all done for them. To what extent does the activities program involve residents in the planning and encourage their participation? Are there physical activities for varying degrees of physical strength and dexterity? Are the intellectual and cultural pursuits open to all who are interested? What are the religious traditions of the establishment? Would you feel comfortable there? What, if anything, would you miss not having available?

Management Philosophy

The philosophy and guiding principles of administration filter down throughout the whole establishment, from the highest official to the newest part-time employee. In interviews, be alert to nuances in the atmosphere of the offices. Do those in authority appear to be in charge without being authoritative? Is there a spirit of cooperation and caring between the office staff and the executive director? If so, this will flow out into the rest of the facility.

Ask about what channels there are for residents to participate in the policies and decisions which directly affect them. Find out if the governing body (this includes the board of directors and the administration) is autonomous or is responsible to a larger organization. Is the executive director there on a full-time basis? Is he or she readily accessible to residents?

Financial Status

Not all continuing care retirement centers are financially stable. Some have gone bankrupt; some have been sold to new management. The financial aspect should be investigated very carefully. Ask for the most recent financial statement of any facility under consideration. If it is hard to understand, a lawyer or accountant can explain it. (For example, a copy of the 1990 financial statement for Foulkeways is included in the appendix of this book. See Appendix B.)

All CCRCs have an entrance fee and a monthly maintenance fee. Some offer a refund to the resident's estate upon his death, in which case the entrance fee is much larger than where there is no refund. Be sure to check into this.

AAHA has a system of rating under their own stringent criteria the facilities they list in the *National Continuing Care Directory*. This is done every five years and is at the request of the CCRC. It involves an extensive self-evaluation by the CCRC, combined with the objective findings of the AAHA examiners. Check the ratings of those in which you are interested.

Armed with this information and the results of your investigations and interviews, you are now able to make an informed and very important decision about what can be some of the most comfortable, contented, and interesting days of your life.

APPENDIX B

SAMPLE FINANCIAL STATEMENT OF FOULKEWAYS AT GWYNEDD

BALANCE SHEET

General Fund	December 31 1990	1989
Assets		
CURRENT ASSETS:		
Cash		
Investments	4,033,188	3,036,619
Accts receivable:		
Residents	767,242	470,908
Other	127,085	87,715
Notes receivable	1,202	3,132
Inventories	39,014	40,418
Prepaid expenses	173,975	133,062
Total current assets	**$5,141,706**	**$3,843,126**
PROPERTY, PLANT AND EQUIPMENT:		
net	**$10,878,760**	**$11,025,963**
ASSETS LIMITED AS TO USE:		
Board-Designated Investments	**$979,401**	**$758,169**
	$16,999,867	**$15,627,258**
Liabilities and Fund Balance		
CURRENT LIABILITIES:		
Current portion of long-term debt	$213,164	$200,780
Accounts payable	325,323	259,645
Accrued salaries and payroll taxes	237,577	227,714
Advanced billings	494,876	453,707
Deferred revenue –nurses' education	18,145	20,971
Total current liabilities	**$1,289,085**	**$1,162,817**
LONG-TERM DEBT:		
less current portion	**$702,429**	**$915,593**
Deferred resident entry fees	**$8,188,088**	**$7,025,812**
advance deposits	**$392,000**	**$392,000**
other liabilities	**$6,683**	**$26,868**
commitments & contingencies	**$6,421,582**	**$6,104,168**
General Fund Balance	**$16,999,867**	**$15,627,258**

RESTRICTED FUNDS	1990	1989
ASSISTANCE FUND:		
Investments	$1,221,540	$1,073,057
Fund balance	$1,221,540	$1,073,057
BUILDING AND EQUIPMENT FUND:		
Investments	$26,528	$24,636
Fund balance	$26,528	$24,636
OTHER RESTRICTED FUNDS:		
Investments	$892,892	$873,356
Fund balance	$892,892	$873,356

STATEMENTS OF REVENUES AND EXPENSES

	December 31	
General Fund	1990	1989
OPERATING REVENUE:		
Resident care revenue	$4,766,238	$4,506,935
Resident entry fee revenue	1,065,575	957,527
Health center revenue –	743,591	757,568
Resident	208,770	197,077
Nonresident	952,361	954,645
Total operating revenue	**$6,784,174**	**$6,419,107**
OPERATING EXPENSES:		
General and administrative	1,065,118	1,050,832
Housekeeping	555,789	512,932
Maintenance	616,046	559,922
Food service	1,547,593	1,489.490
Health center	1,612,330	1,383,190
Utilities	694,443	647,056
Real estate taxes	161,175	148,980
Depreciation	692,839	640,734
Interest expense	61,520	73,185
Total operating expenses	**$7,006,853**	**$6,506,321**
Loss from operations	**($222,679)**	**($87,214)**
NONOPERATING REVENUE:		
Unrestricted contributions, gifts and bequests	23,191	463,252
Investment income	367,146	264,164
Other nonoperating revenue	149,756	138,990
Total nonoperating revenue	540,093	866,407
EXCESS OF REVENUE OVER EXPENSES	$317,414	$779,192

APPENDIX C

HISTORICAL CHRONOLOGY OF FOULKEWAYS PROPERTY

1681	Charles II granted Pennsylvania to William Penn.
3/23/1681	William Penn granted 10,000 acres to Robert Turner.
3/10/1698	Robert Turner by deed poll conveyed 7,820 acres to William John and Thomas ap Evans, yeomen, who named it Gwynedd, meaning high ground.
4/3/1698	Cadwallader Evans, wife and three children, left Fron Goch, Merionethshire in Wales to take ship in Liverpool.
4/18/1698	Ship *Robert and Elizabeth*, Ralph Williams, Master, sailed for the new world via Dublin, Ireland.
7/17/1698	*Robert and Elizabeth* docked in Philadelphia eleven weeks after leaving Dublin.
11/1698	Cadwallader Evans, wife, and their remaining son, John, settled in new home on tract purchased in Gwynedd. House on site now occupied by Hollingsworth mansion.
6/5/1699	William John and Thomas ap Evans deeded 609 acres of land in Gwynedd to Cadwallader Evans for 32 pounds 10 shillings sterling.
1700	First log meetinghouse built at Gwynedd.
1712	Second meetinghouse of stone built on same site.
11/22/1714	Monthly Meeting established at Gwynedd.
3/30/1745	Cadwallader Evans died at Gwynedd, leaving all property to his son, John.
6/22/1757	John Evans died leaving various bequests of land with life tenure but residual interest in main tract to his son, John, with power of bequest.

11/6/1807	John Evans, son of John and Eleanor (above) married Margaret Foulke, daughter of Evan and Ellen Foulke of Gwynedd.
1815	John Evans Estate sold and subdivided several times. The present 68 acre tract was purchased by Dr. Joseph Meredith, who, leaving no issue, bequeathed it to his partner, Dr. Antrim Foulke.
1817	Beaumont House built by blacksmith Morgan, who later expanded.
1823	Present meetinghouse built at Gwynedd.
10/23/1825	Henry Foulke, son of Antrim and Letitia Foulke, born at Gwynedd, married Maria L. Banks in 1852.
6/16/1856	May Foulke, daughter of Henry and Maria Foulke, born at Gwynedd, later married Charles O. Beaumont.
After 1915	Blacksmith shop redesigned by Edwin Brumbaugh into a home.
11/25/1945	Charles O. Beaumont died, bequeathing the property to Gwynedd Friends Meeting as a memorial to his wife, May Foulke Beaumont.

(This chronology was bound into a notebook of Foulkeways papers. We do not know the original source.)

APPENDIX D

GLOSSARY OF QUAKER EXPRESSIONS

Chace Fund — a fund established by Anna H. and Elizabeth M. Chace to be used for religious, charitable or educational organizations.

Chandler Fund — a Quaker fund established to assist nursing homes.

First-Day School — Sunday School.

A concern — something which should be done.

Laid down the committee — discontinued it.

Leading — a sense of direction, Divinely inspired.

Shoemaker Fund — a fund established by Thomas H. and Mary Williams Shoemaker to be used for educational and religious concerns.

Weighty Friend — highly respected person.

Philadelphia Yearly Meeting — parent body of Quarterly Meetings, which are made up of Monthly Meetings in a certain geographical area.

Quarterly Meeting — business meeting held quarterly of constituent Monthly Meetings.

Monthly Meeting — monthly business meeting of local Meeting.

Yearly Meeting — Annual business meetings usually held in the spring and over a period of several days.

Representative Meeting — a committee to handle concerns and business of the Yearly Meeting between the annual sessions.

APPENDIX E

QUAKERS FOR WHOM BUILDING CLUSTERS WERE NAMED

Antrim, Dr. Antrim Foulke (1793–1861). Grandfather of May Foulke.

Barclay, Robert (1648–1690). Early Quaker missionary.

Cadbury. Well-known name in early Quaker history.

Dewsbury, William (1621–1688). A contemporary of George Fox.

Evans, Cadwallader. Original owner of land where Foulkeways was built.

Fox, George, (1624–1688). Founder of Religious Society of Friends. (Quakers).

Greenleaf. J. Greenleaf Whittier (1807–1892). Called the Quaker poet.

Heath, Robert & Susanna. Came to America in 1701.

Jenkins, J.J. Early settlers in Gwynedd. Came from Wales in 1729.

Kendal. Important town for Quakers in England.

Logan, James (1674–1751). Came to Pennsylvania with Wm. Penn.

Mott, Lucretia (1793–1880). Anti-slavery activist.

Norris, Isaac (1671–1735). Came to Philadelphia in 1692.

Pickett, Clarence (1884–1965). Director of American Friends Service Committee for 22 years.

Rowntree, John W. (1868–1905). Founded Woodbrooke, a Quaker study center in England.

Sprogell, Harry. (1912–1972). Prime mover of Foulkeways and vice-president, 1968–1971.

Walton, George (1883–1969). Headmaster, George (Friends) School, 1912–1948.

White, Allen (1912– 1989). Executive Director of Foulkeways, 1967–1989.

Woolman, John (1720–1772). Author of Quaker classic, *The Journal of John Woolman.* Anti-slavery activist.

(continued)

Names of wings in Health Center:

Abington House. Named for the Abington Friends Home in Norristown.
Gwynedd House. Named for Gwynedd, Pennsylvania.
Lloyd Wing. Named for Thomas Lloyd, Quaker physician. Came to Pennsylvania in 1683.
Owen Wing. Named for Griffith Owen, Quaker physician who came to Philadelphia with William Penn.

Information obtained from a paper, *Quaker Background of Foulkeways Names* filed with Foulkeways records.

APPENDIX F

LIST OF FOULKEWAYS BOARD MEMBERS OFFICERS OF THE BOARD ASSOCIATION MEMBERS

Association Members
August 1964 – January 1974

Bartram, Anna S
Braxton, Nina P.
Brunner, Robert B.
Clarke, Eleanor S.
Deibler, Lorraine W.
Evans, Joseph S., II
Foulke, Eliza A.
Hallowell, Charles K.
Hankin, Martha P.
Jacobson, Barbara S.
Martin, August L.
Martin, Marion W.
Osterkamp, Ann L.
Ritchie, Russell W.
Shultz, Agnes, D.
Sprogell, Barbara S.
Stees, Helen G.
Stott, W. Russell
Tobieson, Florence B.
Trueblood, Arnold E.
Trueblood, Caroline F.
Williams, James W., III
Willis, Elizabeth P.
Wright, Lowell E.
Zimmerman, C. Edward

Board Members

Alden, James C., M.D.
Auf der Heyde, Ethel

Baer, John E.
Bartram, Howard
Baumgartner, Steven.
Bennett, Asia A.
Benton, Frederic E.
Bicking, Jeanetta M.
Blackstone, Agnes W.
Blumberg, Grace R.
Brown, Patricia A.
Buckman, F. Preston

Camp, William P.
Clarke, Eleanor S.
Cooper, Dorothy N.

Dickinson, W. Haines, Jr.

Elkinton, Thomas W.
Evans, J. Morris
Ewing, Charles H.

Glenn, Georgie
Goulding, Esther S.

Hallowell, Dorothy B.
Harned, William H.
Henderson, Rolland H.
Hetzel, Millie
Hunt, Alan, Esq.

Jacobs, William J.
Jacobson, Barbara S.

Landry, Lawrence
Lippincott, H. Mather, Jr.
Lockyer, Charles W., Jr.

Maris, Albert B.
Martin, August R.
Martin, Marion W.
Mohan, Reba H.
Moon, Donald L.

Nepley, Katharine C.

Paton, Linda C.
Potts, Jane M.

Pye, William M.

Rhoads, Donald V.
Ritting, Elizabeth

Schmidt Marshall
Sprogell, Harry E.
Stees, Helen G.
Strumpf, Neville E.
Swansen, Samuel T.

Trueblood, Arnold E.
Tweddale, Douglas
Tyndall, George I.

Walker, Tacy E.
Walton, Lewis B., Jr.
Weaver, Thurston L.
White, Allen J.
Willis, Richard B.
Winde, Norman H.

Ziegler-Driscoll, Genevra
Zimmerman, Blanche P.
Zimmerman, C. Edward

Foulkeways at Gwynedd
Current and Former Board Members Holding Offices

PRESIDENT

Winde, Norman 1968–1974
Willis, Richard 1975–1985
Swansen, Samuel 1986–1992

(continued)

VICE PRESIDENT

Sprogell, Harry 1968–1971
Camp, William 1972–1982
Pye, William 1983
Swansen, Samuel 1984–1985
Rhoads, Donald 1986–1989
Buckman, F. Preston 1990–1992

SECRETARY

Stees, Helen 1968–1973
Jacobson, Barbara 1974–1984
Dickinson, W. Haines, Jr. 1985–1987
Moon, Donald 1988–1989
Tweddale, Douglas 1990–1992

TREASURER

Willis, Richard 1968–1974
Lockyer, Charles, Jr. 1975–1980
Landry, Lawrence 1981–1983
Tyndall, George 1984–1992

ASSISTANT SECRETARY

Willis, Richard 1971–1974
White, Allen 1974–1977
Lockyer, Charles, Jr. 1975–1979
Moon, Donald 1978–1988
Tweddale, Douglas 1988–1990

ASSISTANT TREASURER

Sprogell, Harry 1968–1971
Martin, August 1968–1981
Camp, William 1972–1977
Baer, John 1978–1982
Swansen, Samuel 1983
Pye, William 1984–1988
Bartram, Howard 1989
Trueblood, Arnold 1990–1991
Willis, Richard 1992

11/04/91

APPENDIX G

FOULKEWAYS ORGANIZATIONAL STRUCTURE

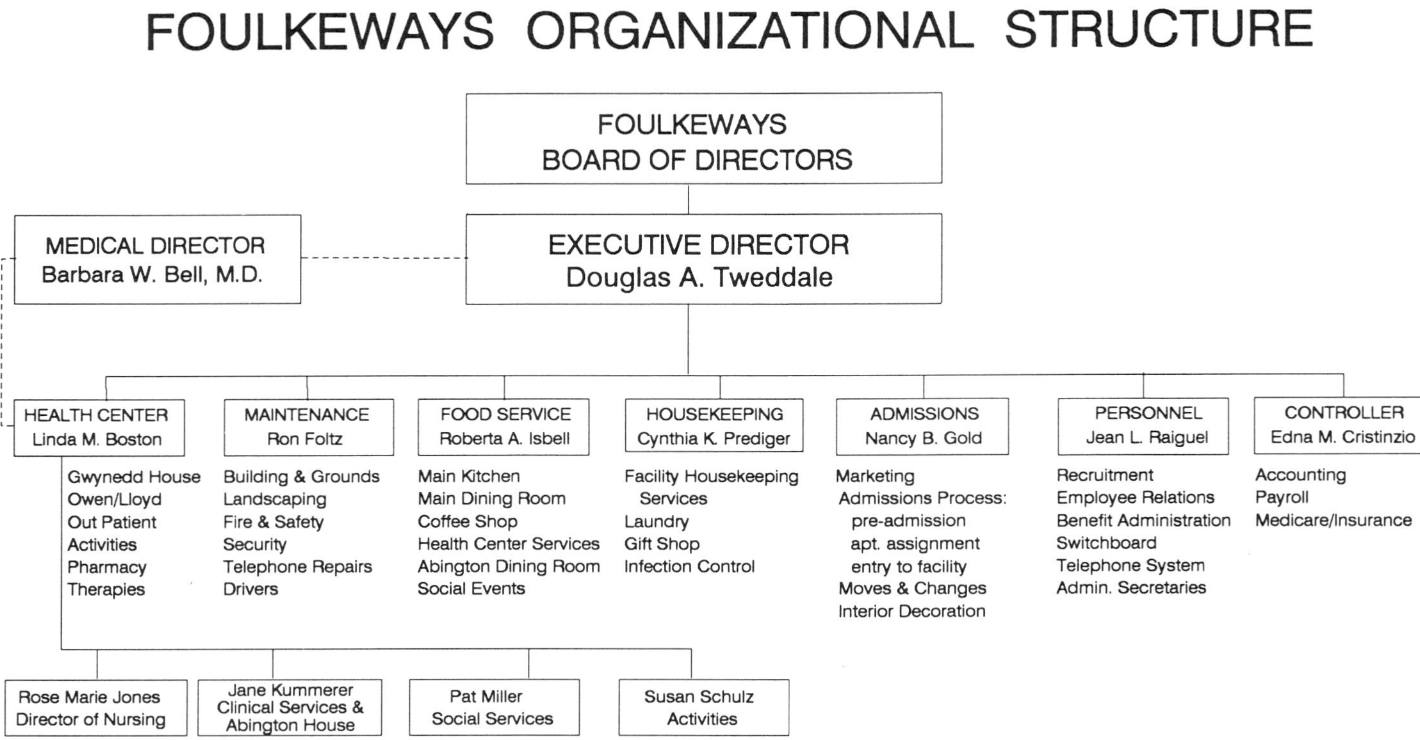

Index of Surnames

INDEX OF SURNAMES

ABOUT THE AUTHOR

Blanche Zimmerman, with her husband, Edward, moved to Foulkeways the first of January, 1988 leaving the farm which had been owned and farmed by Zimmermans since 1775. Blanche, a registered nurse, was graduated from the Lankenau Hospital Training School for Nurses, Philadelphia, Pennsylvania, in 1931 and received a B.A. from Gwynedd-Mercy College, Gwynedd Valley, Pennsylvania, in 1987. They have two children, five grandchildren and four great-grandchildren.

While Blanche has contributed several articles to periodicals, this is her first book.

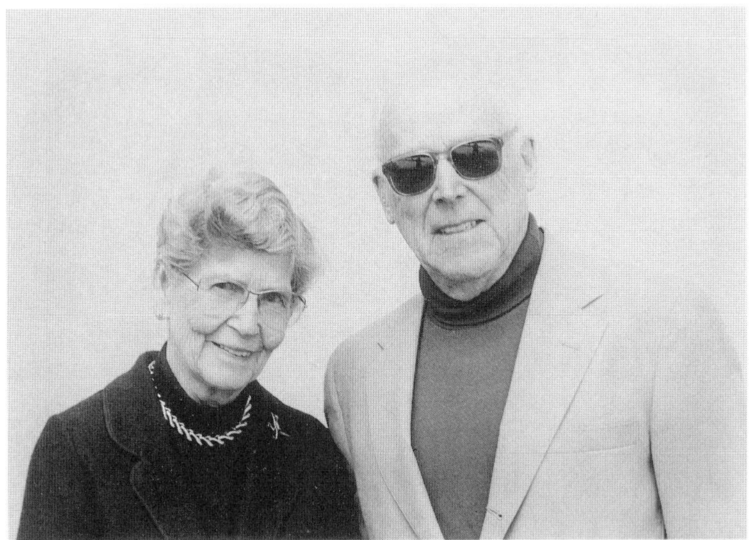

Blanche P. and C. Edward Zimmerman